International Outcome Measures
in Mental Health

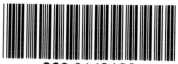

International Outcome Measures in Mental Health

Quality of life, needs, service satisfaction, costs and impact on carers

Graham Thornicroft, Thomas Becker, Martin Knapp, Helle Charlotte Knudsen, Aart Schene, Michele Tansella and José Luis Vázquez-Barquero

Gaskell

Gaskell is an imprint of the Royal College of Psychiatrists,
17 Belgrave Square, London SW1X 8PG

Gaskell is a registered trademark of the Royal College of Psychiatrists.

Photocopying and translation

The material that appears on pages 48–51, 57–58, 77–82, 99–111, 131–138 and 158–169 may be photocopied by individual researchers or clinicians for their own use without seeking permission from the publishers.

Please contact the publishers if you wish to translate any material in this book into another language.

British Library Cataloguing-in-Publication Data

A catalogue record for this book is available from the British Library.

ISBN 1-904671-00-4

Distributed in North America by Balogh International, Inc.

The views presented in this book do not necessarily reflect those of the Royal College of Psychiatrists, and the publishers are not responsible for any error of omission or fact.

The Royal College of Psychiatrists is a registered charity (no. 228636).
Printed in the UK by Cromwell Press Ltd, Trowbridge, Wiltshire

Contents

Acknowledgements

The following colleagues contributed to the EPSILON Study. Amsterdam: Dr Maarten Koeter, Karin Meijer, Dr Marcel Monden, Professor Aart Schene, Madelon Sijsenaar, Bob van Wijngaarden; Copenhagen: Dr Helle Charlotte Knudsen, Dr Anni Larsen, Dr Klaus Martiny, Dr Carsten Schou, Dr Birgitte Welcher; London: Professor Thomas Becker, Dr Jennier Beecham, Liz Brooks, Dr Daniel Chisholm, Gwyn Griffiths, Julie Grove, Professor Martin Knapp, Dr Morven Leese, Dr Paul McCrone, Sarah Padfield, Professor Graham Thornicroft, Dr Ian R. White; Santander: Andrés Arriaga Arrizabalaga, Sara Herrera Castanedo, Dr Luis Gaite, Andrés Herrán, Modesto Perez Retuerto, Professor José Luis Vázquez-Barquero, Elena Vázquez-Bourgon; Verona: Dr Francesco Amaddeo, Dr Giulia Bisoffi, Dr Doriana Cristofalo, Dr Rosa Dall'Agnola, Dr Antonio Lasalvia, Dr Mirella Ruggeri, Professor Michele Tansella.

This study was supported by the European Commission BIOMED–2 Programme (Contract BMH4-CT95-1151). Thanks are due to Dr J. Oliver for his permission to include the Lancashire Quality of Life Profile in the EPSILON Study and for his helpful comments and assistance in its administration and scoring. We would also like to acknowledge the sustained and valuable assistance of the users, carers and the clinical staff of the services in the five study sites. In Amsterdam, the EPSILON Study was partly supported by a grant from the Nationaal Fonds Geestelijke Volksgezondheid and a grant from the Netherland Organization for Scientific Research (940-32-007). In Santander the EPSILON Study was partially supported by the Spanish Institute of Health (FIS) (FIS Exp. No. 97/1240). In Verona additional funding for studying patterns of care and costs of a cohort of patients with schizophrenia were provided by the Regione del Veneto, Giunta Regionale, Ricerca Sanitaria Finalizzata, Venice (Grant No. 723/01/96 to Professor M. Tansella).

Contributors

Francesco Amaddeo	Department of Psychiatry, University of Verona, Italy
Andrés Arriaga Arrizabalaga	Clinical and Social Psychiatry Research Unit, Department of Psychiatry, University of Cantabria, Santander, Spain
Thomas Becker	Department of Psychiatry II, University of Ulm, Germany
Daniel Chisholm	Centre for the Economics of Mental Health, Institute of Psychiatry, King's College London, UK
Doriana Cristofalo	Department of Medicine and Public Health, Section of Psychiatry, University of Verona, Italy
Rosa Bruna Dall'Agnola	Department of Medicine and Public Health, Section of Psychiatry, University of Verona, Italy
Luis Gaite	Clinical and Social Psychiatry Research Unit, Department of Psychiatry, University of Cantabria, Santander, Spain
Thomas Greenfield	Alcohol Research Group, Public Health Institute, Department of Psychiatry, University of California, San Francisco, California, USA
Gwyn Griffiths	Section of Community Psychiatry (PRiSM), Institute of Psychiatry, King's College London, UK
Andrés Herrán	Department of Psychiatry University Hospital Marques de Valdecilla, University of Cantabria, Santander, Spain
Peter Huxley	Health Services Research Department, Institute of Psychiatry, King's College, London, UK
Martin Knapp	Centre for the Economics of Mental Health, Institute of Psychiatry, King's College London and London School of Economics, London, UK
Helle Charlotte Knudsen	Institute of Preventive Medicine, Copenhagen Hospital Corporation, Copenhagen University Hospital, Copenhagen, Denmark
Maarten Koeter	Department of Psychiatry, Academic Medical Centre, Amsterdam, The Netherlands
Antonio Lasalvia	Department of Medicine and Public Health, Section of Psychiatry, University of Verona, Italy
Morven Leese	Section of Community Psychiatry (PRiSM), Institute of Psychiatry, King's College London, UK
Paul McCrone	Section of Community Psychiatry (PRiSM), Centre for the Economics of Mental Health, Institute of Psychiatry, King's College London, UK
Jo Oliver	School of Psychiatry and Behavioural Science, University of Manchester, Manchester, UK

Sarah Padfield	Section of Community Psychiatry (PRiSM), Institute of Psychiatry, King's College London, UK
Modesto Perez Retuerto	Clinical and Social Psychiatry Research Unit, Department of Psychiatry, University of Cantabria, Santander, Spain
Mirella Ruggeri	Department of Medicine and Public Health, Section of Psychiatry, University of Verona, Italy
Aart Schene	Department of Psychiatry, Academic Medical Centre, Amsterdam, The Netherlands
Dolors Serrano López	Department of Psychiatry, University Hospital Marques de Valdecilla, University of Cantabria, Santander, Spain
Deirdre Sierra-Biddle	Department of Psychiatry, University Hospital Marques de Valdecilla, University of Cantabria, Santander, Spain
Mike Slade	Section of Community Psychiatry, Health Services Research Department, Institute of Psychiatry, King's College London, UK
Michele Tansella	Department of Medicine and Public Health, Section of Psychiatry, University of Verona, Italy
Graham Thornicroft	Section of Community Psychiatry, Health Services Research Department, Institute of Psychiatry, King's College London, UK
José Luis Vázquez-Barquero	Clinical and Social Psychiatry Research Unit, Department of Psychiatry, University of Cantabria, Santander, Spain
Elena Vázquez-Bourgon	Clinical and Social Psychiatry Research Unit, Department of Psychiatry, University of Cantabria, Santander, Spain
Birgitte Welcher	Hvidovre Hospital, Department of Psychiatry, Copenhagen Hospital Corporation, Copenhagen University Hospital, Copenhagen, Denmark
Ian R. White	Medical Statistics Unit, London School of Hygiene and Tropical Medicine, London, UK
Bob van Wijngaarden	Netherlands Institute of Mental Health and Addiction, Utrecht, The Netherlands

Part I

Development of scales to measure mental health outcomes

1 The EPSILON Study: aims, outcome measures, study sites and patient sample

Thomas Becker, Martin Knapp, Helle Charlotte Knudsen, Aart H. Schene, Michele Tansella, Graham Thornicroft, José Luis Vázquez-Barquero and the EPSILON Study Group

The development and translation of assessment instruments in mental health is a complex process, which becomes increasingly important in a uniting Europe. The major aim of the European Commission BIOMED-funded multi-site study, the European Psychiatric Services: Inputs Linked to Outcome Domains and Needs (EPSILON) Study, was to produce standardised versions in several European languages of instruments measuring five key concepts in mental health service research (Becker *et al*, 1999): (a) the Camberwell Assessment of Need (CAN), measuring needs for care; (b) the Involvement Evaluation Questionnaire (IEQ), assessing family or care-giving impact; (c) the Verona Service Satisfaction Scale (VSSS), measuring satisfaction with services; (d) the Lancashire Quality of Life Profile (LQoLP), assessing the quality of life of service users; and (e) the Client Socio-demographic and Service Receipt Inventory (CSSRI), assessing service utilisation and costs.

Aims

The outcomes translation, adaptation and reliability assessments presented in this book were part of a wider research project. This is a comparative cross-sectional study of the care of people with schizophrenia in five European countries. Six research teams in five centres were involved, located in Amsterdam, Copenhagen, London (Centre for the Economics of Mental Health and Section of Community Psychiatry, Institute of Psychiatry), Santander and Verona. The centres had experience in health services research and instrument development, and all had access to mental health services providing care for local catchment areas.

The instruments used assess a variety of dimensions of the care process, such as needs for care, service utilisation and costs, informal carer involvement, quality of life and service satisfaction. These research scales were used to study care for people with schizophrenia in five centres cross-sectionally in a sample of patients in contact with secondary mental health services. The EPSILON Study aimed: (a) to produce standardised versions of five key research instruments in five languages; (b) to compare data about social and clinical variables, mental health care and costs; and (c) to test instrument-specific and cross-instrument hypotheses. Facilitating future cross-national research into care for the severely mentally ill is a central objective of the EPSILON Study.

Study instruments

Five study instruments were adapted for use in the five languages and different service settings:

(a)   Camberwell Assessment of Need (CAN);
(b)   Client Service Receipt Inventory (CSRI);
(c)   Involvement Evaluation Questionnaire (IEQ);
(d)   Lancashire Quality of Life Profile (LQoLP);
(e)   Verona Service Satisfaction Scale (VSSS).

These instruments are designed to assess a variety of dimensions of the care process; some of their characteristics are outlined in Table 1.1.

Patients' needs

The European version of the CAN (CAN–EU), an interviewer-administered instrument, was used to assess patients' needs. It is described fully in Chapter 4. It comprises 22 individual domains of need (accommodation, food, household skills, self-care, occupation, physical health, psychotic symptoms, information about condition and treatment, psychological distress, safety to self, safety to others, alcohol, drugs, company of others, intimate relationships, sexual expression, child care, transport, money, welfare benefits, basic education and telephone).

Service use and cost

The Client Socio-demographic and Service Receipt Inventory – European Version (CSSRI–EU) is an adaptation of the CSRI (Beecham & Knapp, 1992) which, on the basis of an interview, records socio-demographic data, accommodation, employment, income, and all health, social, education and criminal justice services received by a patient during the preceding 6 months (Chapter 8). It allows costing of services received on the basis of unit cost data.

Caregiving consequences

The IEQ measures the consequences of psychiatric disorders for relatives of patients (Schene & van Wijngaarden, 1992). The European version (IEQ–EU) contains five sections: general information on the patient, caregiver and household (15 items); caregiving consequences (31 items); costs (8 items); the General Health Questionnaire (GHQ–12); and the consequences for patients' children (11 items). The time frame is the past 4 weeks. Caregiving consequences are summarised using four scales (tension, worrying, urging, supervision) and a summary score (Chapter 10).

Quality of life

The European version of the LQoLP (LQoLP–EU) elicits objective quality of life indicators and subjective quality of life appraisal through patients' answers to interviewer-administered questions relating to nine fields: work/education, leisure/participation, religion, finances, living situation, legal and safety, family relations, social relations and health (Chapter 13).

Table 1.1 Core study instruments

Instrument	No. of domains	No. of facets/ sub-scales explored	No. of items	Mode of administration	Average completion time (mins)	Time frame	Sub-scale score	Summary score	Type of response scale	Presence of manual	Degree of training required
CAN–EU	22	–	22 x 6	INT	20–30	Past month	Yes (met needs, unmet needs, total needs)	Yes	Categorical ratings for presence of need and level of help	Yes	Moderate
CSSRI–EU	5	–	110	INT	20–30	Past 6 months	Yes, 5 service use domains	Various	Categorical and structured responses	Yes	Modest
IEQ–EU	5	4 sub-scales and one total score	31 IEQ; 81 all modules	SA QU	10 min IEQ; 20–30 min for whole set	Past 4 weeks	Yes, 4 + GHQ	Yes	Likert, 5-point (never to always)	No manual needed as IEQ contains instructions	None
LQoLP–EU	9	Positive and negative affect, affect balance	105	INT	30	Past week, month or year (varies)	Yes	Yes	Yes/no, Likert, 7-point	Yes	Little
VSSS–EU	7	7	63	SA[1]	20–30	Past year	Yes, one for each domain	Yes	Likert 5-point	Yes	None/little

1. Assisted in some places:

EU, European Version; CAN, Camberwell Assessment of Need; CSSRI, Client Socio-demographic and Service Receipt Inventory; IEQ, Involvement Evaluation Questionnaire; LQoLP, Lancashire Quality of Life Profile; VSSS, Verona Service Satisfaction Scale; GHQ, General Health Questionnaire; INT, interview-administered; SA, self-administered; QU, questionnaire.

Service satisfaction

Satisfaction with services was assessed using an adapted version of the VSSS (VSSS–EU), a self-administered instrument comprising seven domains (global satisfaction, skill and behaviour, information, access, efficacy, intervention and relatives' support) (Chapter 16).

Other instruments

Other instruments used included the Brief Psychiatric Rating Scale (BPRS 24-item version; Ventura *et al*, 1993) and Global Assessment of Functioning (GAF; American Psychiatric Association, 1987). These were used in English. Instruments documenting the sampling process (Prevalence Cohort Data Sheet), area socio-demographic descriptors (Area Socio-Demographic Data Sheet) and patients' psychiatric history (Psychiatric History Data Sheet) were developed for the EPSILON Study. Descriptions of site-level characteristics included socio-demographic area descriptors, availability of in-patient beds and other service components, and staff availability. The European Service Mapping Schedule was also used (Johnson *et al*, 1998; Becker *et al*, 2002). Data were collected for the EPSILON Study during the period September 1997 to August 1998.

Study sites

Amsterdam

General area characteristics

Data were collected in Amsterdam South-East, which is a 30-year-old borough in the south of the city. It is mainly a residential area, with a mixed lower- and middle-class population of 110 000. Unemployment is high. Fifty per cent of the inhabitants are from one of the 60 minority ethnic groups. Data were collected for 1 January 1998.

Mental health services in the local area

The mental health services in the Amsterdam South-East catchment area are in a process of change and integration, and this paragraph describes the services in January 1998 (during the period of the study). The large Santpoort mental hospital, located 25 km to the west of Amsterdam, during the 1990s started to provide services (out-patient, in-patient and residential) across the city. Having moved to Amsterdam, these services, formerly hospital-based, are now in the process of integrating with mental health services which have been available in the city for many years, such as the Regional Institute for Ambulatory Mental Health Care (Regionale Instelling voor Ambulante Gestelijke Gezordheilzorg, RIAGG) and the Department of Psychiatry at the Academic Medical Centre (AMC).

Since 1998 these three organisations (Santpoort, RIAGG and AMC) have been merged into one organisation called De Meren, with three separate services, for people aged over 65, 18–64, and below 18 years. For the adult population this new organisation offers out-patient services in three locations: the former RIAGG, the out-patient department formerly at Santpoort, and the AMC out-patient department. These three services have been merged into the Social Psychiatric Service Centre (SPSC). This SPSC has its in-patient units (eight beds on a closed ward, six beds on an open intermediate care ward, 20 beds on an open ward) in the AMC, where a 24-hour emergency room is also available. For long-term patients, non-acute 24-hour staffed residential services and sheltered accommodation are available within the SPSC. Services for the catchment area population also include intensive home care, two shelters for homeless people with mental illness, a day care centre and a vocational rehabilitation centre. The wider context of mental health services in Amsterdam is described in more detail elsewhere (Schene *et al*, 1998; Becker *et al*, 1999).

Copenhagen

General area characteristics

Copenhagen is the capital of Denmark, with a total population of about 480 000. Copenhagen is divided into 14 social districts (boroughs). The two neighbouring social districts of Vesterbro and Kongens Enghave were the catchment areas for the project, with a population of about 50 000.

Mental health services in the local area

The mental health services in Vesterbro and Kongens Enghave are provided by Hvidovre Hospital. The psychiatric department of this hospital has an emergency unit with 4 beds, and 130 in-patient beds distributed across three locked wards, three open wards, one ward for young people with first-episode psychosis, one ward open Monday to Friday (each with 15 beds), and an old age psychiatry ward with 10 beds. They provide an extensive liaison psychiatric service to the general hospital. Further, Hvidovre Hospital has three community mental health centres (CMHCs): Vesterbro, Valby and Vanløse. Vesterbro Community Mental Health Centre provides services for inhabitants in the catchment areas Vesterbro and Kongens Enghave (population about 50 000) with chronic mental illness, mostly schizophrenia. Hvidovre Hospital's total catchment area is 130 000. The CMHC has a multidisciplinary team: psychiatrist, psychologist, social workers, nurses, occupational therapist and physiotherapist. The total number of staff is 22. Every patient has a case manager and a psychiatrist in the CMHC. At any one time, approximately 300 patients are on the CMHC case-load. The CMHC provides out-patient care, structured day activities (mostly workshops as social training: arts, cooking, gymnastics and psycho-education) and home visits to patients. The CMHC and the psychiatric department at the general hospital collaborate in setting up different types of conferences, educational programmes, etc. There is close collaboration between the CMHC and other services in the catchment area, such as general practitioners, social services, sheltered accommodation and voluntary organisations (Kastrup, 1998; Becker *et al*, 1999).

London (Croydon)

General area characteristics

Croydon is a predominantly suburban borough in south London, with a total population of 330 000. The population ranges from the somewhat deprived inhabitants of the north of the borough to the more affluent, middle-class residents of the semi-rural southern area. Patients in this study were recruited from a sector population of about 80 000 in the borough.

Mental health services in the local area

Specialist mental health services in Croydon are purchased by Croydon Health Authority and provided by the Bethlem & Maudsley NHS Trust. These specialist mental health services for the general adult population include 70 acute adult psychiatric beds for the 330 000 population; 10 low-security in-patient places in a locked ward; and four medium-security forensic beds. Residential provision includes 25 places staffed around the clock by nurses, 166 places staffed around the clock by other care workers and 22 less well supported places. For the provision of community mental health services, the borough is divided into three localities, and sampling in this study was from the central locality, with a population of about 80 000. Each of these three localities contains two or three general adult community mental health teams, which typically include community psychiatric nurses, an attached social worker, attached occupational therapist, consultant psychiatrist and junior psychiatrist. There are four CMHCs for the whole borough of Croydon. These function as community multidisciplinary team bases, settings for out-patient and depot medication clinics, and as day centres, providing occupational therapy and psychotherapeutic groups. Social services and the private and voluntary sectors also provide day care places, work opportunities and 'drop-in' services (Johnson et al, 1997; Thornicroft & Goldberg, 1998; Becker et al, 1999).

Santander

General area characteristics

The study was conducted in Cantabria, an autonomous community with a population of about 560 000 in northern Spain. Patients were recruited from Cantabria as a whole. The city of Santander, a university town with a total population of about 194 000 inhabitants, is predominantly middle-class, with the majority of those employed working in services and light industry.

Mental health services in the local area

The Spanish Psychiatric Reform, which was formally initiated in 1985, had as its main objective the replacement of the old mental hospitals with alternative services in the community and in-patient psychiatric units in general hospitals (Vázquez-Barquero & García, 1999). These services are integrated in the Spanish National Institute of Health (INSALUD), providing free health care for the whole of the Spanish population. In this context, psychiatric services in Santander are mainly provided as follows:

(a)   There is an acute psychiatric in-patient unit of 42 beds (there are also 12 beds in a long-term psychiatric hospital, used mainly by patients from the private sector, insurance companies and health consortia). This unit, which also meets the needs of the whole region of Cantabria, is located within the Marqués de Valdecilla University Hospital, which is both a teaching general hospital with 1199 beds, providing in-patient services for the region of Cantabria, and a referral hospital for the rest of Spain for tertiary, specialised forms of medical care.

(b)   A 24-hour acute emergency unit is located in the university hospital.

(c)   For the provision of community mental health services, Cantabria is divided into four areas, each with a community mental health service. Santander is one of these mental health service areas: the Santander mental health centre is divided into two multidisciplinary adult mental health teams, each including two psychiatrists, a community nurse, a psychologist and a social worker.

(d)   For long-term psychiatric care, patients can be referred to a long-stay psychiatric hospital belonging to the Cantabria local authorities (114 beds) or to a long-stay psychiatric hospital belonging to a non-profit-making religious organisation (89 beds). Further information is given in Becker et al (1999).

Verona

General area characteristics

Data were collected in the South Verona community-based mental health service (CMHS). South Verona is a predominantly urban area with a population of about 70 000, on the southern outskirts of Verona, a city in northern Italy. Verona is predominantly middle-class, with services and industry constituting more than 90% of the economic sector.

Mental health services in the local area

The South Verona CMHS has developed gradually over the past 20 years, and it is the main psychiatric service providing care to South Verona residents (Tansella et al, 1998). It includes a comprehensive and well-integrated number of programmes, and provides in-patient care, day care, rehabilitation, out-patient care and home visits, as well as a 24-hour emergency service and residential facilities (three apartments and one hostel) for long-term patients. Staff of the CMHS are divided into three multidisciplinary teams, each responsible for a subsector of the catchment area. With the exception of hospital nurses, all staff (psychiatrists, psychologists, social workers and community nurses) work both inside and outside hospital. The 'single staff' module ensures continuity of care through the different phases of treatment and the different components of the service. A Psychiatric Case Register (PCR), which covers the same geographical area, has been operating since 31 December 1978. Private hospitals and other agencies in the larger province of Verona also provide information to the PCR. However, 1990–1993 data indicate that 82% of patients living in the area are receiving care from the South Verona CMHS, either solely or together with other services. The vast majority of patients with a diagnosis of schizophrenia are on the case-loads of public mental health services. It can be assumed that the sample assessed in this study is representative of all patients with a diagnosis of schizophrenia under 'active treatment' in the South Verona catchment area (Tansella et al, 1998; Becker et al, 1999). Data were collected from patients with schizophrenia attending the CMHS in the two 3-month periods October–December 1997 and April–June 1998; this timing was chosen to coincide with routine assessments taking place as part of the South Verona Outcome Project (Tansella et al, 1998; Becker et al, 1999).

Case ascertainment

In this study, adults aged 18–65 inclusive with any ICD–10 diagnosis from F20 to F25 were included at the screening stage. These administrative prevalence samples of patients with psychotic disorders were identified either from psychiatric case registers (in Copenhagen and Verona) or from the case-loads of local specialist mental health services (in-patient, out-patient and community). Patients needed to have been in contact with mental health services during the 3-month period preceding the start of the study. Thus, an administrative prevalence sample of people with schizophrenia in contact with mental health services was used in each site as the sampling frame. Cases identified were diagnosed using the item group checklist (IGC) of the Schedule for Clinical Assessment in Neuropsychiatry (SCAN; World Health Organization, 1992). On this basis, only patients with an ICD–10 F20 research diagnosis were included in the study.

Exclusion criteria included current residence in prison, secure residential services or hostels for long-term patients; coexisting learning disability (mental retardation), primary dementia or other severe organic disorder; and extended in-patient treatment episodes longer than 1 year. This was done in

Table 1.2   Diagnostic distribution in initial sample at screening stage

ICD–10 diagnostic group	Amsterdam n	Amsterdam %	Copenhagen n	Copenhagen %	London n	London %	Santander n	Santander %	Verona n	Verona %
F20 schizophrenia	123	79	100	69	149	86	300	71	84	45
F21 schizotypal disorder	–	–	18	13	9	5	4	1	8	4
F22 persistent delusional disorder	9	6	6	4	–	–	44	10	29	15
F23 acute transient psychotic disorder	–	–	9	6	5	3	52	12	20	11
F24 induced delusional disorder	–	–	–	–	–	–	1	–	1	1
F25 schizoaffective disorder	2	1	5	4	6	4	22	5	17	9
Other	15	10	3	2	4	2	–	–	15	8
No diagnosis	5	4	3	2	–	–	–	–	14	7
Total	154	100	144	100	173	100	423	100	188	100

order to avoid any bias between sites due to variation in the population of patients in long-term institutional care, and to concentrate on those in current 'active' care by specialist mental health teams. The numbers of patients finally included in the study varied from 52 to 107 between the five sites, with a total of 404.

Patient sample

The distribution of diagnoses on the basis of the item group checklist (Table 1.2) shows that between 45% (in Verona) and 86% (in London) of the patients screened had an IGC diagnosis of schizophrenia. Schizotypal disorders were most likely to be diagnosed in Copenhagen (13%); both persistent delusional disorders and acute transient psychotic disorders were more likely to be diagnosed in Santander (10% and 12% respectively) and Verona (15% and 11% respectively) than in the other sites.

Table 1.3 shows the attrition of the samples and reasons why interviews could not be completed. Some differences require comment. The order of events was: (a) collection of administrative data, including all prevalent cases in contact with catchment area services; (b) random selection of patients who were diagnosed and/or interviewed (not in London and Verona, where all were eligible, in order to achieve a big enough sample); (c) diagnostic assessment on the basis of the IGC SCAN (World Health Organization, 1992); and (d) the study interview. In Copenhagen, the matching of prevalent cases and those interviewed was not possible, due to patient confidentiality regulations in the Danish legal and data protection systems. In Amsterdam, London and Verona all (or most) patients were contacted for interview, because large numbers of refusers and patients who could not be found, as

Table 1.3   Sample attrition

	Amsterdam	Copenhagen	London	Santander	Verona	Total
All prevalent cases	170	144[1]	173	423	188	1098
Selected for IGC rating/interview	154		173	125	184	–
Excluded (SCAN or ICG)	31		4	0	42	–
Lost/died/ill/refused/age excluded	62		85	25	35	–
Final data-set	61	52	84	100	107	404

ICG, item group checklist; SCAN, Schedule for Clinical Assessment in Neuropsychiatry.
1. Match between prevalent cases and subsequent screened individuals not possible owing to Danish patient confidentiality regulations (72 excluded altogether).

Table 1.4 Comparisons between those interviewed, and those selected at random and meeting inclusion criteria but not interviewed (excluding Copenhagen)

	Interviewed	Not interviewed[1]	P[2]
Number (maximum[1])	352	203	–
Age (years)	41.2	40.1	0.27
Years since first contact	11.7	11.7	0.95
Total number of contacts	1.96	1.98	0.37
Lifetime psychiatric admissions	4.0	6.3	0.14
Male	57%	59%	0.59
Married	18%	13%	0.21
White	93%	89%	0.26

1. Because lost, ill, died, refused.
2. Data missing for some individual variables.

well as substantial diagnostic heterogeneity, were expected. The proportion of patients excluded on the basis of the IGC diagnosis varied from none (Santander) to high rates of 18% and 22% (Amsterdam, Verona). This may reflect differences either in clinical diagnostic routine or in the case-load composition of the secondary mental health services in the various sites. Patients not located varied from 1% (Santander, Verona) to 16% (London), which may reflect more social integration in the former, and more deprivation and loss of social networks in the latter. The rate of interview refusals varied from 3% (Santander) to 32% (London). Again, Santander and Verona had low rates and contrasted with London, and this might reflect social context and degrees of deprivation or integration. Between 21% (Amsterdam) and 57% (Verona) of patients completed the interview at time 1, and this may reflect differences between recently established (Amsterdam) and long-standing (Verona) community mental health services. Table 1.4 shows comparisons between patients interviewed and those not interviewed; there was no significant difference.

Contents and outlook

This book summarises the EPSILON Study in terms of instrument adaptation (Chapter 2) and psychometric methods applied in testing instrument reliability (Chapter 3). The individual instruments used and adapted in this study are described in detail in Chapters 4, 8, 10, 13 and 16. The output of this process is a set of 'EU' instrument versions available in five languages (Danish, Dutch, English, Italian and Spanish). Data obtained using these instruments provided a multidimensional picture of the needs of people with schizophrenia, their service use and their subjective appraisal of quality of life and services available. By making these instruments available to a wider audience of researchers and service managers involved in mental health services research and planning throughout Europe, it is hoped that they will make a lasting contribution to the field of mental health services research.

References and further reading

American Psychiatric Association (1987) *Diagnostic and Statistical Manual of Mental Disorders* (3rd edn, revised) (DSM–III–R). Washington, DC: APA.

Becker, T., Knapp, M., Knudsen, H. C., et al (1999) The EPSILON Study of schizophrenia in five European countries: design and methodology for standardising outcome measures and comparing patterns of care and service costs. *British Journal of Psychiatry*, **175**, 514–521.

Becker, T., Hülsmann, S., Knudsen, H. C., et al (2002) Provision of services for people with schizophrenia in five European regions. *Social Psychiatry and Psychiatric Epidemiology*, **37**, 465–474.

Beecham, J. & Knapp, M. (1992) Costing psychiatric interventions. In *Measuring Mental Health Needs* (eds G. Thornicroft, C. R. Brewin & J. Wing), pp. 163–183. London: Gaskell.

Johnson, S., Ramsay, R., Thornicroft, G., *et al* (eds) (1997) *London's Mental Health*. Report to the King's Fund London Commission. London: King's Fund.

Johnson, S., Salvador-Carulla, L. & the EPCAT group (1998) Description and classification of mental health services: a European perspective. *European Psychiatry*, **13**, 333–341.

Kastrup, M. (1998) Mental health in the city of Copenhagen, Denmark. In *Mental Health in Our Future Cities* (eds D. Goldberg & G. Thornicroft), pp. 101–123. Hove: Psychology Press.

Oliver, J., Huxley, P., Bridges, K., *et al* (1996) *Quality of Life and Mental Health Services*. London: Routledge.

Schene, A. H. & van Wijngaarden, B. (1992) *The Involvement Evaluation Questionnaire*. Amsterdam: Department of Psychiatry, Academic Medical Center, University of Amsterdam.

Schene, A. H., Hoffmann, E. & Goethals, A. L. J. (1998) Mental health in Amsterdam. In *Mental Health in Our Future Cities* (eds D. Goldberg & G. Thornicroft), pp. 33–55. Hove: Psychology Press.

Tansella, M., Amaddeo, F., Burti, L., *et al* (1998) Community-based mental health care in Verona, Italy. In *Mental Health in Our Future Cities* (eds D. Goldberg & G. Thornicroft), pp. 239–262. Hove: Psychology Press.

Thornicroft, G. & Goldberg, D. (1998) London's mental health services. In *Mental Health in Our Future Cities* (eds D. Goldberg & G. Thornicroft), pp. 15–31. Hove: Psychology Press.

Vázquez-Barquero, J. L. & García, J. (1999) Deinstitutionalization and psychiatric reform in Spain. *European Archives of Psychiatry and Clinical Neuroscience*, **249**, 128–135.

Ventura, J., Green, M. F., Shaner, A., *et al* (1993) Training and quality assurance with the Brief Psychiatric Rating Scale: 'the drift busters'. *International Journal of Methods in Psychiatric Research*, **3**, 221–244.

World Health Organization (1992) *Schedules for Clinical Assessment in Neuropsychiatry* (ed.-in-chief J. K. Wing). Geneva: WHO.

2 Translation and cross-cultural adaptation of outcome measurements for schizophrenia

Helle Charlotte Knudsen, José Luis Vázquez-Barquero, Birgitte Welcher, Luis Gaite, Thomas Becker, Daniel Chisholm, Mirella Ruggeri, Aart Schene, Graham Thornicroft and the EPSILON Study Group

Research on the comparison of mental health services has identified the need for internationally standardised and reliable measures which can describe and compare patients, services, costs and outcomes across language and cultural boundaries. Equivalent language versions of an instrument will make it possible to carry out multi-centre research and make meaningful comparisons of results obtained in different countries (Sartorius & Helmchen, 1981).

Often mental health measurements and psychological tests have been developed for content, validity and reliability in one country or language exclusively. Some of these instruments are then used in other languages and cultural settings, but often without detailed attention to the cross-national and cross-cultural adaptation that is necessary. Few instruments have been produced in equivalent versions in different languages, thus ensuring, in addition to their validity and reliability, their cross-cultural applicability in the new setting (Sartorius & Kuyken, 1994). The methods involved and their difficulties have been well described by different authors (Simonsen & Mortensen, 1990; Sartorius & Kuyken, 1994; Gaite *et al*, 1997; Hutchinson *et al*, 1997).

This chapter describes the process used in the EPSILON Study to translate and adapt five research instruments for cross-cultural use within five European countries – the Camberwell Assessment of Need (CAN), the Client Socio-demographic and Service Receipt Inventory (CSSRI), the Involvement Evaluation Questionnaire (IEQ), the Lancashire Quality of Life Profile (LQoLP) and the Verona Service Satisfaction Scale (VSSS) – and summarises the impact that the methods used had on the development of the instruments. This process included the following steps: (a) translation; (b) cross-cultural verification and adaptation; (c) verification of the psychometric properties of the instrument in the target language. The first two elements of this process are considered in this chapter, which describes in detail the use of focus groups as part of the cross-cultural adaptation process. The third step – verifying the psychometric properties of the instruments – is described in Chapter 3.

Translation approach

Sartorius & Kuyken (1994) describe four approaches to translation of instruments from a source to a target language, depending on the degree of conceptual overlap between the source and the target culture: (a) the ethnocentric approach (100% conceptual overlap); (b) the pragmatic approach (considerable conceptual overlap); (c) the emic plus etic approach (less conceptual overlap); and

(d) translation not possible (when there is no conceptual overlap). 'Conceptual overlap' means the extent to which a concept has the same meaning in both cultures – for example, the concept of 'corruption' has intuitively very different meanings in different parts of the world, as have the concepts of health and illness (Box 2.1).

Box 2.1 Concepts used in the literature describing the translation process

Approaches to the development of cross-culturally applicable questionnaires
(Hutchinson *et al*, 1997)

- Sequential approach: translation and performance evaluation of an existing instrument

- Parallel approach: international conceptualisation of measurement and selection of content

- Simultaneous approach: international conceptualisation of construct around which the cross-national core item set is developed, where each nation or culture develops its own specific content.

Approaches to translation of questionnaires already developed
(Sartorius & Kuyken, 1994)

- Ethnocentric approach: 100% conceptual overlap between source and target culture

- Pragmatic approach: considerable conceptual overlap (for example: European context)

- Emic plus etic approach: some degree of conceptual overlap

- Translation impossible: no conceptual overlap.

Translation and types of equivalence
(Sartorius & Kuyken, 1994; Hutchinson *et al*, 1997)

- Conceptual equivalence: refers to same concepts underlying the questions in both source and target languages (review of cross-cultural literature or factor analysis)

- Semantic equivalence: denotative (what the word indicates or is a sign for) and connotative (what is the primary meaning of the word) sameness; use synonyms to identify the semantic space

- Linguistic equivalence: when the item in the target version has a similar meaning to that in the source version; retaining the functional equivalence. The same as semantic equivalence

- Technical equivalence: equivalence of technical features of the languages and their relationship to the sociocultural context (language complexity, question length, acceptable level of abstraction); and feasibility of the nature and mode of questioning of the instrument in the source and target versions (for example, the method of applying the questionnaire: paper and pencil, or semi-structured or structured interview).

Cross-cultural equivalence

- Content equivalence: when each item of the questionnaire describes a phenomenon relevant to both cultures

- Semantic equivalence: concerned with retaining the meaning of each item

- Conceptual equivalence: the validity of the concepts in both cultures

- Technical equivalence: whether the way in which data collection is carried out affects the result differently in different cultures

- Criterion equivalence: akin to criterion validity, which is an instrument's relationship to independent criteria of the same phenomena.

The translation approach selected depends on the degree of overlap between the source and the target cultures of the concepts in question. In a European context, there is considerable conceptual overlap in most measures regarding patients, services, costs, or outcomes in mental health services; therefore the pragmatic approach is suitable when an instrument developed in Europe is translated into other European languages and cultures.

Within each of these approaches, the aim of translation is to maintain, as far as possible, semantic (or linguistic), conceptual and technical equivalence between the versions of the instruments in the source and target languages (Sartorius & Kuyken, 1994; Hutchinson *et al*, 1997). 'Semantic equivalence' is the retaining of similar meanings of a measure in the source and target versions, whereas 'conceptual equivalence' refers to the need to obtain an identical meaning of concepts that might have different cultural interpretations – for example, the concept of 'good mental health' (Sartorius & Kuyken, 1994; Hutchinson *et al*, 1997). Finally, 'technical equivalence' refers to both the technical features of the languages (i.e. language complexity, question length, acceptable level of abstraction) and their relationship to the sociocultural context (the feasibility of the nature and mode of questioning used in the instrument in the source and target versions; for example: whether the questionnaire is applied as a self-rating questionnaire or as a structured interview). These three equivalencies are the key to a proper translation of instruments. They require those involved in the translation procedures to be highly qualified. Translators should ideally have good technical knowledge of both the source and the target languages, and full emotional understanding of both languages; be deeply involved in the cultures in question; know about the cultural problems related to the concepts and terms used in the questionnaire (so they can, for example, avoid the use of stigmatising concepts); and to have integrated knowledge of the area and domains explored in the questionnaire. In practice, translators will meet these rigorous criteria to varying degrees. When a translator does not have all these characteristics, this can be compensated for by interactive discussions with experts, consultations with monolingual panels not involved in the translation process, or other strategies specifically designed for the translation of health assessment instruments.

However accurate the translation process, it will not necessarily guarantee that the instrument has been fully adapted to the target language, in the sense that the concepts and constructs incorporated in the instrument are fully applicable. To achieve this, specific quantitative and qualitative strategies need to be adopted: for example, concept mapping (Russell, 1988), pile sorting (Trotter & Potter, 1993), key-informant consensus meeting (Johnson, 1990) and focus groups. The focus group method was selected for the EPSILON Study.

Use of focus groups

The focus group interview is a procedure first described by Bogardus (Bogardus, 1926). It was initially used by commercial companies for market research, to develop and evaluate a diverse range of products; to analyse target populations' wishes, views, problems, fears, beliefs and vocabulary; and to shape communication in advertising campaigns. More recently, it has been used in political campaigns and health education programmes, and it has also proved useful in mental health research, by providing qualitative information for both qualitative and quantitative research designs (Room *et al*, 1996).

The focus group interview is a qualitative research method. It is based on the formal group interview, which in its structure and method derives from group psychotherapy, and takes the form of a focused group interview or an arranged talk/communication among a selected group of people. Its aim is to uncover important dimensions of a given problem, experience, service or other phenomenon (Basch, 1987; Krueger, 1994; Bojlén & Lunde, 1995). The advantage of focus groups is that by careful selection of the participants, and by developing the outline of the group session in accordance with the aims of the focus group interview (exploratory, judgemental, phenomenological) (Basch, 1987,

p. 418), we can produce a wide range of information and potentially uncover important understanding of the problem to be addressed. It is possible to address instrument problems such as the readability of a measure, the construct of the concept, or the understanding of the mental health care system, and at the same time address the issue of acceptability of the content of the questions (such as financial, religious or sexual issues).

Basch (1987) has outlined the key features of the focus group interview: the role of the moderator, the physical setting, the psychological climate conducive to a successful session, proper selection of participants in accordance with the aim of the focus group interview, instrumentation (development of discussion outline and questions to be asked), data collection and analysis, including a summary report on the findings.

It is recognised in group psychotherapy that the optimum size for a good working group is six to ten participants, and the size of the group affects the nature of the data collected as well as the group structure. In general, it is thought that focus groups should be highly structured, with six to ten members, and with moderators controlling both the questions to be asked and the group dynamics. This approach is appropriate when the moderator knows what the key questions are.

Developing the discussion outline and the questions to be used by the moderator requires careful thought and a considerable amount of effort in planning. As in all questionnaire design, each item of the outline has a specific purpose. The data obtained in the focus group interview can be analysed in different ways, depending on the method used for data collection (tape recording, videotape, written notes); whichever method is used, the final version of the report should contain a summary outlining the most important ideas and conclusions. Potential problems and technical issues are related to unbiased data reduction and the inferences to be drawn from qualitative data.

Method

Translation protocol

The five instruments selected for the translation and cultural adaptation process all had to be translated into four other languages. A protocol was developed, describing each step in the translation process:

(a) Each instrument was translated from its original language into the target language by a professional translator, who received information on the content of the instrument being translated. The translation from the original language into the target language was made by a translator whose native language was the target language and whose second language was that of the original instrument.

(b) The translator and the research group discussed the first translation. This led to a revision of the translation and a list of disputed translation items.

(c) The translated instrument was then back-translated into the original language by a different translator, whose native language was that of the original instrument and whose second language was the target language. The second translator also commented on the first translation and the list of disputed items.

(d) The back-translation was compared with the original version. Differences were discussed by the first translator and the researchers. This led to another revision of the translation and a list of disputed items to be considered by the focus group in the country concerned.

(e) The focus group's remarks were discussed by the researchers with one of the translators. Inappropriate and impossible items and sentences were revised. This led to the final version.

With some modifications, this procedure was followed for the translation of all five instruments.

Focus group procedure

Running the focus group involved seven main tasks:

(a) Establishing the list of topics to be discussed. The subject for each group was the translated version of the instrument to be adapted. The topics discussed were translation adequacy, instrument applicability and the concepts of the constructs. The centre responsible for each instrument prepared a list of important issues to be discussed by the focus group, based on problems raised during the translation process. In addition to this, group participants could discuss other themes they considered relevant.

(b) Choosing where to hold the focus group. It was important to conduct the sessions in places free from interruption by external activities.

(c) Choosing the participants. The focus group was composed of a moderator (often the group leader), a co-leader and the other participants. The moderator had skills in facilitating effective group functioning and was either a psychiatrist or a psychologist. The co-leader assisted the leader in taking notes of relevant issues during the session, collaborated in the analysis of the group material and provided other perspectives. Six to ten participants were selected for each group, and at each site separate focus groups were set up for each questionnaire. Participants represented the different categories of people involved in the delivery and receipt of care: both men and women; doctors, nurses, social workers, patients, relatives, and also (depending on the instrument in question) local administrators, social workers, general practitioners and psychologists. The composition of the group was decided taking into consideration each of the topics selected for analysis: for example, administrators and social workers were considered important participants in the focus group assessing the CSSRI.

(d) Conducting the focus group session. A specific guideline was developed for each of the instruments, guiding both the questions and the issues to be raised during the session, and the composition of the group; group sessions were highly structured, and lasted for about an hour and a half.

(e) Data collection during the focus group session. The moderator and co-leader took notes at each session; they noted, among other things, the participants, late arrivals, relationships to other participants, the start time, the list of questions asked, the time when each major issue or question was asked; and recorded the major probe questions used and the actual arrangement (seating) of participants in the session. Comments made by the moderators about each person's participation and notes on session processes included, for example, notes on who was speaking, notes on the tone of the session and any problem areas that occurred and how (if at all) they were resolved. The process was recorded differently in each country. In Italy, for example, sessions were videotaped, whereas in Denmark two reporters were included in the group to take the notes.

(f) Post-session data completion. At the end of the focus group session the moderator and the co-leader (plus the reporters) completed the notes taken during the session. The notes included an overall assessment of the session, its strengths and weaknesses, notes on key issues that were raised and notes about individual participants and their contributions, as well as any other useful or relevant information.

(g) Reporting the results of the focus group. The focus group proceedings were reported immediately in the native language, and later the key issues of the report were conveyed in a report in English for discussion in the international research group (Table 2.1).

Table 2.1 Reporting on the focus groups

Selection of participants	
Focus group contact list	All contacts made with the individuals on the initial contact list, including their response to the contact; key characteristics that led to an individual's selection for the group
Data collection during focus group session	
Focus group notes	Record of all focus group participants; note late arrivals, relationships to other participants, etc. The starting time, a list of questions asked, notes of the time when each major question is asked, and a record of major probe questions used and actual arrangement (seating) of participants in the session
Post-session data completion	
Focus group notes	The moderator and any other team members present complete a post-session debriefing and record any potentially useful information about the session

Structure of the report

Under 'Items', the report deals with linguistic problems uncovered during the discussion, opinions about the applicability and relevance of the items, topics arising due to overlapping of items present in different areas of the instrument, and suggestions about items that the participants consider should be included. Under 'Topics' reported a number of general topics in connection with the instrument were discussed by the participants, illustrating differences between participants in the interpretation of different subjects. Reports were designed to:

(a) Isolate the major themes of each focus group in relation to the problems being explored. It is important to recognise categories, themes, issues, and explanations from the descriptions made by the participants in the session.

(b) Ensure that, after the information from the interview had been sorted into categories, it could be compared. This way possible categories or sets of ideas emerging from the data could be identified.

(c) Draw conclusions; once the general pattern had been described, a picture of prevailing beliefs, opinions, attitudes and explanations regarding each particular instrument or area of the instrument was obtained.

Impact of the focus group on instrument development

The results of these strategies for conversion to the different languages and cultures influenced the development of the instruments' concepts and constructs. The developmental process can be categorised as: (a) changes in the instrument structure, contents and concepts; (b) adjustments to the instrument structure; (c) modifications to the instrument manual. In this chapter we summarise the most relevant overall decisions adopted in each of these categories; a more detailed account is given in the chapters describing the individual instruments.

Changes in the instrument structure, contents and concepts

Involvement Evaluation Questionnaire

The Involvement Evaluation Questionnaire was considered by focus groups in Denmark, England, Italy and Spain. The conclusion was that the instrument covered the main domains of family burden well. There were some problems with items regarding education, type of professional help, income categories, and drug use; and the response categories were discussed. The instrument was adjusted in accordance with the comments received; the response categories, however, remained unchanged, because otherwise comparison with earlier research would become difficult. The items on psychological distress were taken out and the General Health Questionnaire, 12-item version (Goldberg & Hillier, 1979) was included to describe general well-being.

Client Socio-demographic and Service Receipt Inventory

The instrument underwent major changes as a consequence of the focus group process in order to enable comparisons to be made between different countries' health care and social welfare systems. The diversity in organisation of the welfare systems in the participating countries made it especially difficult to find a common language in this area of the questionnaire. The many comments from the focus groups were an important contribution to solving these problems. In addition, internationally comparable concepts for describing individual socio-demographic variables were added to the instrument.

Adjustments to the instrument structure

Verona Service Satisfaction Schedule

The Verona Service Satisfaction Schedule was discussed in focus groups in Denmark, England, the Netherlands and Spain. The instrument was considered acceptable in all countries and underwent relatively minor modifications. There were some problems regarding the grouping of professional staff, such as psychiatrists and psychologists, and nurses and social workers, caused by the different structures of the mental health care systems. These problems were solved by asking questions regarding each professional group separately. Issues related to the organisation of health care and social welfare were clarified, and translation issues were taken into consideration.

Modification incorporated in the instrument manuals

Lancashire Quality of Life Profile

The Lancashire Quality of Life Profile was subjected to the focus group process in Denmark, Italy, the Netherlands and Spain, which gave rise to a lengthy discussion regarding its suitability, arising from earlier psychometric analyses of the instrument. All countries agreed that the instrument is the most comprehensive quality-of-life instrument available in the field of mental health services research.

Camberwell Assessment of Need

The Camberwell Assessment of Need was considered by focus groups in Denmark, Italy, the Netherlands and Spain. The overall views were mixed, and there were many suggestions for additional items, although there was consensus on only a small number of such additional items. However, it was decided not to change the instrument as it has already been used in many countries. Instead, the 'missing items' were addressed in a revised manual for the instrument. Translation issues raised through the focus groups led to modifications in each new language version.

Benefits of using focus groups

International comparison of mental health services has made the need for internationally standardised instruments clear. In recent years interest in the problems of translation and cross-cultural adaptation of health and service outcome measures has grown considerably (Simonsen & Mortensen, 1990; Sartorius & Kuyken, 1994; Gaite *et al*, 1997; Hutchinson *et al*, 1997). The main concern in this process is to ensure semantic, conceptual and technical equivalence between the versions of the instrument in different languages (Sartorius & Kuyken, 1994). Meadows *et al* (1997) have suggested that this set of criteria be considered as a minimum in the adaptation and use of instruments in cross-cultural studies, much in line with Sartorius & Kuyken (1994), and add, as an intermediate set of key issues, criterion equivalence and content equivalence (when each item of the questionnaire describes a phenomenon relevant to both cultures); they also suggest the use of focus groups to evaluate the semantic equivalence of the adapted instrument.

In the outline of the focus group interviews for each instrument, we included questions and probes related to an identified list of disputed translated issues (semantic equivalents), the readability of the instrument (technical equivalence) and the construct of the concepts (concept equivalence), in accordance with the minimum criteria described. We included questions to the focus groups regarding the content of instruments: did the items of the questionnaire describe a phenomenon relevant to the culture, and should other items be added to describe relevant phenomena? All instruments were modified to improve semantic and technical equivalence; however, the modifications made to improve conceptual equivalence varied, depending on the extent to which the instrument had already been accepted for use in international research.

To our knowledge, this is the first cross-national study reporting on the use of focus groups as a method in the process of converting instruments into internationally comparable measurements, to assess the semantic, conceptual and technical issues in existing, pre-selected instruments. However, groups of this type are not in general different from other focus groups used to identify thoughts, beliefs and feelings; and this method shares, in general, the same advantages and disadvantages as other qualitative research methods (Trotter, 1991; Room *et al*, 1996).

One of our main concerns in using focus group interviews in instrument development has been the question of the reliability and generalisability of the information gathered. The careful selection of participants, representing different positions in mental health care systems, and also representing different gender and socio-demographic groups, helps to generalise the results. However, only people living in cities participated in the focus groups in this study; we have no information on the extent to which this population is also representative of people living in the rural areas of Europe.

In structured focus group sessions, the moderator has an important role in ensuring that the information gathered is representative of the participants present. The group requires a setting that will encourage a trusting, comfortable and secure atmosphere, so that potentially vulnerable contributors (for example, patients and relatives) do not withdraw themselves from the process; also, it is important to prevent dominant members of the group from determining the content of the discussion. The moderators in the EPSILON Study were trained in group sessions, and were either psychologists or qualified psychiatrists, which we found enabled us to run the groups in a way that encouraged the right atmosphere.

The instruments modified in the EPSILON Study were at different stages of development for international use. The CSSRI's main domains were defined, but the internationally comparable concepts and constructs had yet to be developed (Chapter 8); another instrument, the IEQ, had been used in some European studies, but reconstruction of the sequence of some questions and constructs (the construct of general well-being) was considered to be an important improvement to the instrument and accepted by its developers (Chapter 10). Three instruments, however, were already in frequent use in European research (CAN, LQoLP, VSSS); changes to their concepts and constructs were considered less appropriate by the developers, because the existing form of the instrument was already internationally accepted.

Organising and running focus groups is a time-consuming process, with many participants and many parties involved, both in the groups themselves and in the discussions of their results and reports. It is our experience that this time is well spent if the instruments are still in their developmental phase, or have seldom been used internationally: in these situations, focus groups contribute information about concepts, constructs and language that is crucial to the development of the instruments for international application. For instruments already used extensively in international research, and where major changes in the instruments are considered less appropriate, focus groups bring less benefit. Most of the improvements in these instruments were related to semantic and technical equivalence; less time-consuming methods of targeting these problems – such as monolingual panels and expert groups – should be considered.

Summary

During the focus group sessions we obtained valid information about the problems we wanted to be discussed. The focus group interview was a structured and creative process, producing information on the applicability of the instruments in different cultures and different health care systems. The extent to which instruments were adjusted in accordance with group reports varied; as an alternative to changing the instrument, sometimes comprehensive manuals were developed to clarify problems that might arise in their use. Based on our experience using focus groups, we suggest that researchers involved in the process of developing instruments for international use first consider:

(a) to what extent the instrument in question is already used in international research;
(b) to what extent changes in the concepts and constructs of the instrument are acceptable to the instrument's developers;
(c) the choice of appropriate methods that specifically target the issues in question.

The use of focus groups is appropriate if concepts, constructs and translation issues are to be addressed. Otherwise, less time-consuming methods should be considered.

References and further reading

Basch, C. E. (1987) Focus group interview: An underutilized research technique for improving theory and practice in health education. *Health Education Quarterly*, **14**, 411–448.

Beecham, J. & Knapp, M. (1992) Costing psychiatric interventions. In *Measuring Mental Health Needs* (eds G. Thornicroft, C. R. Brewin & J. Wing), pp. 163–183. London: Gaskell.

Bogardus, E. S. (1926) The group interview. *Journal of Applied Sociology*, **10**, 372–382.

Bojlén, N. S. & Lunde, I. L. (1995) Focusgruppeinterview som kvalitativ forskningsmetode. (Focus group interview as a qualitative research method.) *Ugeskrift for Laeger*, **157**, 3315–3318.

Gaite, L., Ramirez, N., Herrera, S., et al (1997) Traducciæn y adaptaciæn y transcultural de instrumentos de evaluaciæn en psiquiatria: aspectos metodolægicos. *Archivos de Neurobiologica*, **60**, 91–111.

Goldberg, D. & Hillier, V. F. (1979) A scaled version of the General Health Questionnaire. *Psychological Medicine*, **9**, 139–145.

Hutchinson, A., Bentzen, N. & Kînig-Zahn, C. (1997) *Cross Cultural Health Outcome Assessment: A User's Guide* (Vol. 1). European Research Group on Health Outcomes.

Johnson, J. C. (1990) *Selecting Ethnographic Informants*. Newbury Park, CA: Sage.

Krueger, R. A. (1994) *Focus Groups: A Practical Guide for Applied Research*. London: Sage.

Meadows, K., Bentzen, N. & Touw-Otten, F. (1997) Cross-cultural issues: an outline of the important principles in establishing cross-cultural validity in health outcome assessment. In *Cross Cultural Health Outcome Assessment: A User's Guide* (eds A. Hutchinson, N. Bentzen & C. Kînig-Zahn), Vol. 1, pp. 34–40. European Research Group on Health Outcomes.

Oliver, J. (1991) The Social Care Directive: development of a quality of life profile for use in community services for the mentally ill. *Social Work and Social Sciences Review*, **3**, 5–45.

Room, R., Janca, A., Bennett, L. A., *et al* (1996) WHO cross-cultural applicability research on diagnosis and assessment of substance use disorders: an overview of methods and selected results. *Addiction*, **91**, 199–220.

Russell, B. H. (1988) *Research Methods in Cultural Anthropology*. London: Sage.

Sartorius, N. & Helmchen, H. (1981) Aims and implementation of multi-centre studies. *Modern Problems of Pharmacopsychiatry*, **16**, 1–8.

Sartorius, N. & Kuyken, W. (1994) Translation of health status instruments. In *Quality of Life Assessment in Health Care Settings* (eds J. Orley & W. Kuyken), Vol. 1. Berlin: Springer.

Simonsen, E. & Mortensen, E. L. (1990) Difficulties in translation of personality scales. *Journal of Personality Disorders*, **4**, 290–296.

Trotter, R. T. I. (1991) Ethnographic research methods for applied medical anthropology. In *Applied Medical Anthropology* (ed. C. Hill), pp. 172–203. Washington, DC: American Anthropological Association.

Trotter, R. T. I. & Potter, J. M. (1993) Pile sorts, an anthropological model of drug and AIDS risks for Navajo teenagers: assessment of a new evaluation tool. *Drugs and Society*, **7**, 23–39.

3 Methodology of a multi-site reliability study

Aart Schene, Maarten Koeter, Bob van Wijngaarden, Helle Charlotte Knudsen, Morven Leese, Mirella Ruggeri, Ian R. White, José Luis Vázquez-Barquero and the EPSILON Study Group

Throughout Europe there is a trend away from hospital-based services towards a variety of locally based community care services for people with severe mental health problems. These community-based services are likely to be better at targeting services to the needs of the most disabled patients, and, as a consequence, are more likely to produce better outcomes at lower treatment and social costs. However, they are organisationally more complex, and potentially more demanding on the families of the patients and the local communities. This organisational complexity makes community care difficult to evaluate. Proper evaluation of these newer forms of service requires a multidimensional approach (Knudsen & Thornicroft, 1996), which, in addition to assessing the usual patient characteristics of psychopathology and social functioning, should focus on concepts such as need for care, satisfaction with services, quality of life, and family or caregiving burden. To measure these concepts, several instruments have been developed in Europe during the past decade (Schene, 1994; Tansella, 1997). Although some have been translated into other European languages, in most cases their cultural validity and reliability have not been adequately assessed. In an attempt to rectify this omission, the EPSILON Study produced standardised versions in five European languages (Danish, Dutch, English, Italian and Spanish) of the Camberwell Assessment of Need (CAN), the Client Socio-demographic and Service Receipt Inventory (CSSRI), the Involvement Evaluation Questionnaire (IEQ), the Lancashire Quality of Life Profile (LQoLP) and the Verona Service Satisfaction Scale (VSSS). These research instruments were developed in three steps: (a) translation and back-translation according to World Health Organization standards into the five European languages, as described in Chapter 2; (b) a review of the translations by the focus group technique (Chapter 2); and (c) evaluation of the instruments' reliability in the five European cultural settings, which is the subject of this chapter (see also Schene *et al*, 2000; Leese *et al*, 2001).

Reliability: theoretical considerations

The quality of any measurement instrument (such as an interview or questionnaire) depends on the validity and reliability of the instrument. 'Validity' refers to the extent to which a (test) score matches the actual construct it has to measure, or in other words to the bias or impact of systematic errors on test scores. 'Reliability' refers to the extent to which the results of a test can be replicated if the same individuals are tested again under similar circumstances, or, in other words, to the precision and reproducibility or the influence of unsystematic (random) errors on the test scores.

Two approaches to reliability can be distinguished: modern test theory (item response theory) and classical test theory. The item response approach makes a comparison of an instrument's performance over different populations possible because, contrary to classical test theory, reliability coefficients in item response theory are not influenced by the population variance. This advantage, however, is diminished by the assumptions concerning the quality of data (e.g. monotonically increasing tracelines, local independence of the items, and – in most cases – dichotomous items), limiting the applicability of an item response approach to those relatively scarce data that fulfil these constraints. In addition, a large number of respondents at each site (200–1000) is needed for an item response approach. The constraints on the data, as well as the sample size requirements, made the item response approach not feasible for the EPSILON Study (Donner & Eliasziw, 1987), and it was therefore decided to base the reliability analyses in this study on classical test theory.

In classical test theory, a person's observed score can be expressed as $X_i = T_i + E_i$, where X_i is the observed score, T_i the true score and E_i the error or random, non-systematic part of the score. In psychology and psychiatry, 'gold standards' are lacking, and so the true score is defined as the theoretical average score over an infinite number of administrations of the same test. Given the assumptions of classical test theory, the variability in the observed scores in a group of respondents (σ^2_X) is composed of the variability in their 'true' scores (σ^2_T) and an error component (σ^2_E). The reliability of a test (ρ_{XX}) is defined as the ratio between true score variance and observed score variance (σ^2_T / σ^2_X). Test reliability defined in the 'classical' way therefore depends to a large extent on the true score variance of the population in which the test was originally developed (since $\sigma^2_X = \sigma^2_T + \sigma^2_E$). If the test is used in another population with a different true score variance (for instance, it might have a lower variance because this population is more homogeneous with respect to the construct under study) the reliability will become lower. For example, in a sample where the error component (σ^2_E) is 0.10 and the true score variance (σ^2_T) is 40, reliability will be 0.80. In another sample with the same error component of 10 but a true score variance of 20, reliability will be 0.66. This 'population' dependence of the reliability coefficient makes comparisons between populations tricky. Differences in reliability between two populations can be caused by differences in precision of the instrument between the populations under study (σ^2_E), or by differences in true score variance of the populations under study (σ^2_T).

One way of handling this problem is the use of the standard error of the mean (s.e.)$_m$, which equals the error component of variance (σ_E). The (s.e.)$_m$, unlike a reliability coefficient, is independent of the true score variance ((s.e.)$_m$ = (s.d.)$_x \sqrt{(1 - \rho_{XX})}$, where (s.d.)$_x$ is the standard deviation between subjects). The (s.e.)$_m$ can be interpreted in two ways. First, it can be used to indicate limits within which the observed score would be expected to lie. For example, if the true score were 10, and the (s.e.)$_m$ were 5, for 68% of the time one would expect the observed score to lie in the range 5–15. Second, it indicates the difference to be expected on retesting or between two raters. For example, if the first observed score were 10, the second observed score would be expected to lie in the range 2.9–17.1 ($10 \pm \sqrt{2} \times 5$) for 68% of the time. The (s.e.)$_m$ is therefore particularly useful when assessing the precision of an instrument in absolute terms, in relation to an individual measurement.

Importance of reliable instruments

The reliability of instruments is of importance for at least two reasons.

(a)   Low reliability automatically implies low validity. The reliability of a measure is defined as the squared correlation between the observed score X and the true score T ($r_{XX} = r^2_{XT}$), a correlation which in the case of perfect reliability equals 1. The validity of a measure is defined as the correlation between the true score, T, and the construct one wants to measure, Y. If the validity is perfect, the true score is identical to the actual construct ($T = Y$). Differences between observed scores and Y are only caused by random errors (and hence $r_{XY} = r_{XT} = \sqrt{r_{XX}}$). In this case the validity coefficient equals the square root of the reliability coefficient. If validity is not perfect, the value of the validity coefficient will be lower than the square root of reliability; so the reliability coefficient sets the upper limit for the validity coefficient ($r_{XT} \leq \sqrt{r_{XX}}$).

(b) Unreliability masks the true relationship between constructs under study. If the error components of the observed scores are uncorrelated, the maximum theoretical possible correlation between two unreliable measures is the square root of the product of their respective reliabilities: $r_{X1X2} \leq \sqrt{r_{X1X2}r_{X1X2}}$). So research for relationships between different constructs is seriously hampered by unreliable operationalisations of these constructs.

Reliability assessment procedures

In this study three different reliability measures are used, depending on the nature of the instruments involved and the way they are administered (interviews v. questionnaires): (a) Cronbach's α for scales and sub-scales consisting of more than one item; (b) Cohen's κ to estimate the interrater reliability and test–retest reliability of single items; and (c) the intraclass correlation coefficient (ICC) to estimate the interrater reliability and test–retest reliability of scales and sub-scales.

Cronbach's α

If a particular construct is measured by means of a scale consisting of two or more items, measures of internal consistency can be used to estimate the reliability of the scale. A simple measure of internal consistency is the split-half reliability of a scale, obtained by randomly dividing the scale into two sub-scales and calculating the correlation between those two sub-scales. The Cronbach's α statistic can be considered as the average of all possible split-half reliabilities of a scale. It is sometimes referred to as the internal consistency coefficient (Streiner & Norman, 1995). However, one should take into account that α is a function not only of the mean inter-item correlation (a real measure of the internal consistency) but also of the number of items of the scale; hence an increase in α does not automatically mean an increase in the internal consistency. Therefore α can more properly be interpreted as the lower limit of the proportion of variance in the test scores explained by common factors underlying item performance (Crocker & Algina, 1986), such that the lower limit of the reliability – the 'true' reliability – is at least as high as α (Dunn, 1989).

The value of α may be expected to substantially underestimate the reliability if different items measure different quantities (Shrout, 1998); as, for example, in the CAN, where differences between needs in different areas reduce the value of α but do not necessarily imply poor reliability. On the other hand, the errors in individual items in the same scale at the same time may well be positively correlated, which will tend to inflate α relative to the reliability.

Interrater reliability

Compared with self-report data, interview data have an additional source of variance that may account for lack of consistency: the interviewer. Although one would prefer an interview, when administered by two different interviewers to the same patient, to produce approximately the same scores – under the assumption that the patient has not changed over time – this is not always the case. Standardisation and structuring of the interview, combined with a thorough training, should in practice diminish the influence of any idiosyncratic characteristics of the interviewers.

The generalisability of the interview scores over interviewers can be estimated by computing a measure of interrater reliability which quantifies the extent to which the information obtained by a specific interviewer can be generalised to other (potential) interviewers. Cohen's κ coefficient is used for categorical data in this study (for variables with more than two categories, a weighted version of the κ coefficient can be used), and ICC for data with at least an ordinal level of measurement.

Strictly speaking, κ is a measure of agreement, not a reliability coefficient, since it is not defined as a ratio of true score variance to observed score variance. Kappa is defined as $(P_o - P_e)/(1 - P_e)$, where P_o is the observed agreement and P_e is the chance agreement: a value of 0 means that the observed agreement is exactly what could be expected by chance; a value of 1 indicates perfect agreement.

The ICC is computed as the ratio of between-patient variance to total variance, which is the sum of between-patient variance and error variance (Streiner & Norman, 1995). If systematic bias is present (for example, if one rater systematically reports higher scores than the other), then this is reflected in the ICC.

Test–retest reliability

The test–retest reliability coefficient, sometimes called the stability coefficient, tests the assumption that when a characteristic is measured twice, both measures must lead to comparable results. However, test–retest reliability is only a valid indicator of the reliability of an instrument if the characteristic under study has not changed in the interval between testing and retesting. This means either a relatively stable characteristic (such as intelligence, personality or socio-economic status) or a short time interval. A short interval between test administrations, however, may produce biased (inflated) reliability coefficients, due to the effect of memory.

Crocker & Algina (1986) ask two questions with regard to the interpretation of a stability coefficient as a measure of reliability. First, does a low value of the stability coefficient imply that the test is unreliable or that the construct itself has changed over time? Second, to what extent is an examinee's behaviour or perception of the situation altered by the test administration? In the EPSILON Study we are dealing with relatively stable constructs, so low stability will indicate low reliability. However, some effect of the test administration on a patient's behaviour and/or perception cannot be ruled out. For this reason, the value of the stability coefficient must be considered as a lower limit for the test–retest reliability.

As was the case with interrater reliability, the kind of test–retest statistics used in this study depends on the nature of the instruments. In the case of items containing categorical data (weighted) κ is used. In the case of instruments containing ordinal scales and sub-scales, the ICC statistic is used.

Interviewer characteristics may cause systematic differences between test and retest interview scores. Although reliability, strictly speaking, only refers to unsystematic differences, we believe that the interviewer-related systematic differences should also be taken into account when evaluating the test–retest reliability of the instruments. For this reason we do not use statistics insensitive to systematic change, such as rank order correlations, but κ and ICC.

Design and procedure of the reliability analysis

Study sites

For this study, researchers from five centres geographically and culturally spread across the European Union (Amsterdam, Copenhagen, London, Santander and Verona) joined forces. All had experience in health services research, mental health epidemiology, and the development and cross-cultural adaptation of research instruments, and had access to mental health services providing care for local catchment areas.

Sample

The EPSILON Study sample was composed of people aged between 18 and 65 years inclusive with an ICD–10 diagnosis of schizophrenia (code F20), in contact with mental health services during the 3-month period preceding the start of the study. Exclusion criteria and case ascertainment are detailed in Chapter 1. For the test–retest reliability analysis, a randomly selected subsample of patients were tested twice within an interval of 1–2 weeks. The sample sizes differed between sites, ranging from 21 to 77 for the IEQ and from 46 to 81 for the LQoLP (see Chapters 4, 8, 10, 13 and 16 for more detailed information).

Core study instruments

The assessment of needs was made using the European versions of the CAN (CAN–EU). The CAN–EU is an interviewer-administered instrument comprising 22 individual domains of need. The IEQ–EU is an 81-item instrument which measures the consequences of psychiatric disorders for relatives of the patient; caregiving consequences are summarised in four scales: tension, worrying, urging and supervision. The VSSS–EU is a self-administered instrument comprising seven domains: global satisfaction, skill and behaviour, information, access, efficacy, intervention and relatives' support. The LQoLP–EU is an interview that assesses both objective and subjective quality of life on nine dimensions: work/education, leisure/participation, religion, finances, living situation, legal and safety, family relations, social relations and health. The CSSRI–EU is an interview in which socio-demographic data, accommodation, employment, income and all health, social, education and criminal justice services received by a patient during the preceding 6 months are recorded. It allows costing of services received after weighting with unit cost data. (The complete instruments and their development are described in Chapters 4, 8, 10, 13 and 16.)

Reliability protocol

To compare the results from the reliability analyses for the different instruments, a strict protocol was developed (Schene *et al*, 1997) to ensure that all centres used the same procedure and options, and the same software, to test the reliability of instruments and to compare the reliability results of the different centres. The protocol covered the following aspects: definition of the specific reliability measures used; description of the statistical methods to assess these reliability coefficients; development of statistical programmes to make inter-centre reliability comparisons; criteria for good reliability; criteria for pooling v. not pooling data; and the general format for the reliability analysis. In Table 3.1 the reliability estimates used are presented for all instruments. The justifications for these estimates for each instrument are given in the relevant chapters of this book.

Statistics

Reliability estimates Cronbach's α was computed for each site, using the Statistical Package for the Social Sciences reliability module (SPSS 7.5 or higher). Intraclass correlation coefficients were computed using the SPSS general linear model variance components option with maximum likelihood estimation in SPSS. Patients were entered as random effects, and in the case of pooled estimates, the centre was entered as fixed effects. Variance estimates were transformed into ICC estimates with corresponding standard errors using an Excel spreadsheet, inputting the between-patient and error components of

Table 3.1   Reliability testing for each instrument

Instrument	Score distribution: mean & s.d. tests	Internal consistency		Test–retest reliability[1]				Systematic change: paired t-test
		α	α test	κ	κ test	ICC	ICC test	
CAN								
Items				*				
Sumscore	*	*	*			*	*	*
LQoLP								
Scales	*	*	*			*	*	*
Sumscore	*	*	*			*	*	*
IEQ								
Scales	*	*	*			*	*	*
Sumscore	*	*	*			*	*	*
VSSS								
Items				*	*			
Scales	*	*	*			*	*	*
Sumscore	*	*	*			*	*	*

CAN, Camberwell Assessment of Need; LQoLP, Lancashire Quality of Life Profile; IEQ, Involvement Evaluation Questionnaire; VSSS, Verona Service Satisfaction Scale.
An asterisk (*) indictates that the reliability assessment is complete.
1. Also interrater reliability for CAN.

variance and their variance-covariance matrix, the latter being used to obtain standard errors based on the delta technique (Dunn, 1989). Unweighted κ estimates were computed using the SPSS module 'crosstabs', weighted κ using STATA version 5.0 (Statacorp, 1997). The standard error of measurement for a (sub-)scale is computed by substituting Cronbach's α for ρ_{xx} in the formula for the $(s.e.)_m$ given earlier (for α) or directly from the error component of variance (for ICCs).

Inter-site comparisons Tests for differences in α values between sites were performed using the Amsterdam α-testing program ALPHA.EXE (Wouters, 1998, based on Feldt *et al*, 1987). Homogeneity of variance between sites was tested with Levene's statistic. For all scales and sub-scales, Fisher's Z transformation was applied to ICCs to enable approximate comparisons to be made between sites (Donner & Bull, 1983). Differences between sites were tested for significance by the method of weighting (Armitage & Berry, 1994) before transforming back to the ICC scale. The standard error of measurement was obtained from the 'error' component of variance.

Finally, a paired *t*-test on test–retest data was carried out in order to assess systematic changes from time 1 to time 2. For the separate items of the CAN, test–retest reliability and interrater reliability for each site were computed as pooled κ coefficients. For the separate items of the VSSS, weighted κ values were computed by site and summarised into bands.

Reliability criteria

For a psychological test, standards used for good reliability are often α ≥0.80, ICC ≥0.90 and κ ≥0.70. The instruments in this study, however, are not psychological tests, like (for instance) a verbal intelligence test. The constructs they cover are more diffuse than in psychological tests and the boundaries with other constructs (such as unmet needs and quality of life) are less clear. As a consequence, the items constituting these (sub-)scales are more diverse and less closely related than would be the case in a strict, well-defined one-dimensional (sub-)scale. Taking these points into consideration, applying the 'psychological test' standards for good reliability to our instruments seems somewhat unrealistic. Landis

& Koch (1977) give some benchmarks for reliability, with 0.81–1.0 termed 'almost perfect', 0.61–0.8 'substantial' and 0.41–0.60 'moderate'. Shrout (1998) suggests revision of these descriptions so that, for example, 0.81–1.0 would be 'substantial' and 0.61–0.80 would be 'moderate'. However, taking account of the special nature of the data in this study, one can consider 0.5–0.7 as 'moderate', and 0.7 and over as 'substantial', and these descriptions have informed the discussion of the adequacy of the coefficients.

Pooled v. separate analysis

In a multi-site study such as this, there are many reasons why one might wish to combine data from the different sites: to summarise the reliability analyses, to identify comparable patients in different sites, and to obtain a larger sample for regression analyses. Whether combining data is reasonable depends on the aim of the analysis and on the results of the reliability analysis for each site.

A first aim is to summarise the level of reliability in the study as a whole. Computing a pooled estimate of a reliability coefficient is reasonable if the site-specific coefficients do not differ significantly. Otherwise a pooled estimate would obscure the variations – but, subject to this proviso, it might nevertheless provide a useful summary.

A second aim is to make comparisons between patients from different sites with the same scale scores: for example, in order to compare outcomes between sites adjusted for differences in symptom severity. This requires scale scores for symptom severity to have the same meaning in different sites. Unfortunately the reliability analysis is unable to tell us whether this is the case. Even with perfect reliability, site A might consistently rate the same actual severity higher than site B; yet this might not be apparent from the data if the mean severity was lower in site A.

A third aim of pooling the samples is to have a larger sample on which to conduct correlation or regression analyses. The possibility discussed above (that sites may differ systematically) makes it desirable that these analyses should adjust for site. Differences in reliability are also important in this case. Lack of reliability in outcome variables will decrease precision, and where this differs between sites, weighting might be necessary. For explanatory variables, there is the more serious problem of bias due to their unreliability, which again might differ between sites. These 'untoward effects' of inefficiency and bias are vanishingly small when reliability is moderate (Shrout, 1998), but one would nevertheless wish to ensure that apparent differences between sites were real, and not just due to these effects. A possible solution for the bias problem is to use 'errors in variables' regression, which can adjust for the effects of differing reliabilities at each site. Analyses should, strictly speaking, be carried out on the type of patients for whom reliability has been established. In the present study, the reliability study was nested within the large substantive study, and the inclusion criteria were similar across sites, so there should be no major problem here.

Analysis scheme

For all instruments the following analysis scheme was followed:

(a) assessment of site-specific reliability estimates – α, ICC, $(s.e.)_m$;
(b) test for inter-site differences in reliability estimates;
(c) test for inter-site differences in score distribution – mean and variance (analysis of variance, and Levene test).

In addition to the site-specific analyses, pooled reliability estimates were made. Where all estimates are high (say, above 0.9), then small differences in reliability between sites may be statistically significant, yet relatively unimportant in practical terms. However, where reliability is generally lower, or lower for one or more sites, differences in reliability between sites imply that pooled estimates should be treated with great caution. In such cases, it is necessary to extend the inter-site comparisons with a consideration of the site (s.e.)$_m$ values, differences in underlying score distributions, and possible reasons for differences: for example, in the way in which the instrument was applied. Furthermore, any imprecision and bias due to such differences would also need to be taken into account in the analysis of pooled data, in the ways mentioned above.

For the CSSRI–EU a different approach was chosen, because it is a new instrument developed for use in a European setting. Since it is an inventory of socio-economic indicators and service variables rather than a multi-item rating scale, the focus was on achieving validity rather than formal reliability (for more details see Chapter 8).

Conclusion

Many technical issues surround the choice of measures of reliability. Such measures are tools which indicate, among other things, the degree to which associations between variables may be diluted; and poor reliability indicates a problem with an instrument when used to quantify associations. Although good reliability does not necessarily indicate a good instrument, reliability studies are one of the best means available to validate our translated instruments.

References and further reading

Armitage, P. & Berry, G. (1994) *Statistical Methods in Medical Research* (3rd edn). Oxford: Blackwell Scientific.

Becker, T., Knapp, M., Knudsen, H. C., *et al* (1999) The EPSILON Study of schizophrenia in five European countries: design and methodology for standardising outcome measures and comparing patterns of care and service costs. *British Journal of Psychiatry*, **175**, 514–521.

Beecham, J. & Knapp, M. (1992) Costing psychiatric interventions. In *Measuring Mental Health Needs* (eds G. Thornicroft, C. R. Brewin & J. Wing), pp. 163–183. London: Gaskell.

Crocker, L. & Algina, J. (1986) *Introduction to Classical and Modern Test Theory*. New York: Holt, Rinehart & Winston.

Donner, A. & Bull, S. (1983) Inferences concerning a common intraclass correlation coefficient. *Biometrics*, **39**, 771–775.

Donner, A. & Eliasziw, M. (1987) Sample size requirements for reliability studies. *Statistics in Medicine*, **6**, 441–448.

Dunn, G. (1989) *Design and Analysis of Reliability Studies*. London: Edward Arnold.

Feldt, L., Woodruff, D. & Salih, F. (1987) Statistical inference for coefficient alpha. *Applied Psychological Measurement*, **11**, 93–103.

Knudsen, H. C. & Thornicroft, G. (1996) *Mental Health Service Evaluation*. Cambridge: Cambridge University Press.

Landis, J. R. & Koch, G. G. (1977) The measurement of agreement for categorical data. *Biometrics*, **33**, 159–174.

Leese, M. N., White, I. R., Schene, A. H., *et al* (2001) Reliability in multi-site psychiatric studies. *International Journal of Methods in Psychiatric Research*, **10**, 29–42.

Oliver, J. (1991) The social care directive: development of a quality of life profile for use in the community services for the mentally ill. *Social Work & Social Sciences Review*, **3**, 5–45.

Oliver, J., Huxley, P., Priebe, S., *et al* (1997) Measuring the quality of life of severely mentally ill people using the Lancashire Quality of Life Profile. *Social Psychiatry and Psychiatric Epidemiology*, **32**, 76–83.

Phelan, M., Slade, M., Thornicroft, G., *et al* (1995) The Camberwell Assessment of Need: the validity and reliability of an instrument to assess the needs of people with severe mental illness. *British Journal of Psychiatry*, **167**, 589–595.

Ruggeri, M. & Dall'Agnola, R. (1993) The development and use of the Verona Expectations for Care Scale (VECS) and the Verona Service Satisfaction Scale (VSSS) for measuring expectations and satisfaction with community-based psychiatric services in patients, relatives and professionals. *Psychological Medicine*, **23**, 511–523.

Sartorius, N. & Kuyken, W. (1994) Translations of health status instruments. In *Quality of Life Assessments: International Perspectives* (eds J. Orley & W. Kuyken), pp. 19–32. Berlin, Heidelberg: Springer.

Schene, A. H. (1994) *Report of the First International ENMESH Conference: Mental Health Service Evaluation: Developing Reliable Measures*. Amsterdam: Department of Psychiatry, Academic Medical Centre, University of Amsterdam.

Schene, A. H. & van Wijngaarden, B. (1992) *The Involvement Evaluation Questionnaire*. Amsterdam: Department of Psychiatry, Academic Medical Centre, University of Amsterdam.

Schene, A., Koeter, M. & van Wijngaarden, B. (1997) *Assessing Needs and Cost-Effectiveness of Care for People Severely Disabled by Schizophrenia in the EU: Reliability Protocol.* Amsterdam: Department of Psychiatry, Academic Medical Centre, University of Amsterdam.

Schene, A. H., Koeter, M., van Wijngaarden, B., *et al* (2000) Methodology of a multi-site reliability study. The EPSILON study of schizophrenia in five European countries 3. *British Journal of Psychiatry,* **177** (suppl 39), 15–20.

Shrout, P. E. (1998) Measurement reliability and agreement in psychiatry. *Statistical Methods in Medical Research,* **7**, 301–307.

Statacorp (1997) *Stata Statistical Software Release 5.0.* College Station, TX: Stata Corporation.

Streiner, D. & Norman, G. (1995) *Health Measurement Scales: A Practical Guide to their Development and Use.* Oxford: Oxford University Press.

Tansella, M. (ed.) (1997) Making Rational Mental Health Services. *Epidemiologia e Psichiatria Sociale,* Monograph Supplement 1. Rome: Il Pensiero Scientifico Editore.

Vázquez-Barquero, J. L. & Gaite, L. (1996) *Focus Group Interview. Final Protocol.* Santander: Clinical and Social Psychiatry Research Unit, University of Cantabria.

World Health Organization (1992) *Schedules for Clinical Assessment in Neuropsychiatry* (ed.-in-chief J. K. Wing). Geneva: WHO.

Wouters, L. (1998) *Amsterdam Alpha-testing Program.* ALPHA.EXE. Amsterdam: Academic Medical Centre.

Part II

Camberwell Assessment of Need – European Version

4   Introduction and manual for the CAN–EU

Paul McCrone, Mike Slade, Morven Leese, Graham Thornicroft, Gwyn Griffiths and the EPSILON Study Group

The Camberwell Assessment of Need – European Version (CAN–EU) is a tool for the comprehensive assessment of the needs of people with severe mental illness. It acts as a filter to highlight areas that might require further detailed assessment: for example, if housing is shown as a need, a housing officer might be asked to carry out a full assessment. The CAN–EU rates met and unmet needs. It is designed for use without prior training, by professionals who have had practice in assessment interviews but have no specific area of expertise. The CAN–EU includes the views of both the service user and the staff member, typically the user's keyworker. Thus differing perceptions of need are accommodated, and specific assessments will take account of both user needs and professional judgement. The time scale of assessment is the preceding month, and this relatively short time span leads to a snapshot assessment of what may be a changeable situation. Adminstration typically takes 15 min per user and 10 min per staff member. One way of using this assessment would be to incorporate it into a 6-monthly review or individual care plan. The original British version of the Camberwell Assessment of Need was developed at the Institute of Psychiatry, King's College London, by Mike Slade, Michael Phelan, Graham Dunn, Frank Holloway, Geraldine Strathdee, Graham Thornicroft and Til Wykes.

Completing the CAN–EU

The CAN–EU contains 22 topics, each of which is divided into four sections. The questions refer to the person's circumstances during the past month, and this time scale should be emphasised in the interview. The interviewer can be the keyworker or another member of staff. The staff rating boxes on each page are completed to reflect the keyworker's perception about the person's need in each area. If the service user is well enough to be interviewed, the user rating boxes are also completed, so that the interview results in a single document containing comprehensive assessments by both the service user and the staff member.

If the service user has difficulties with conversation, it is helpful to allow regular breaks during the interview, perhaps with less demanding conversation. Each topic is self-contained, and it is best to try to finish a topic before having a break. It may be necessary to complete the assessment over more than one session, but the CAN–EU is short enough that this should not often be necessary. In different European settings item 19 (telephone) may not be relevant; if this is the case, then this item can be left unanswered. Item 5 (daytime activities) should also take account of sports and leisure activities.

It is the interviewee's perception of need that is rated, even if the interviewer disagrees with this perception.

The order in which the questions are asked can vary depending on the particular interview. It is not essential that you start with accommodation needs and finish with benefits.

Section 1

The purpose of Section 1 is two-fold. First, it is a filter to decide the appropriateness of further questions for this topic. Second, it records whether effective help is already being given. Suggested opening questions are given in italics. If other questions are thought to be more appropriate for gathering the required information, then these should be used. The examples given may not always be applicable, and therefore it may be more appropriate to use nationally specific examples.

The rating scale for each topic is 0, no problem; 1, no problem, or moderate problem with help given; 2, serious problem; 9, not known. The rating is made using the following algorithm:

- if a serious problem is present (regardless of any help given), rate 2;
- if there is no serious problem *because of help given*, rate 1;
- otherwise rate 0;
- if the respondent does not know or does not want to answer questions on this topic, rate 9.

A need can exist for a variety of reasons. For example, someone with a psychotic illness might be unable to do their own shopping because they are unable to carry it. They should be rated as having a need in the 'food' section, even though this needs is not related to their psychiatric condition.

If someone was an in-patient during the previous month but has what the patient considers to be adequate accommodation outside the hospital, then Section 1 of the 'accommodation' topic will be rated as 0, even though the patient is currently being provided with accommodation. This is an example of 'over-met need', which the CAN–EU does not assess. Over-met need is equated with having no need.

If the rating is 1 or 2 (the person had a need in this area in the past month), then ask the questions in Sections 2–4 on the same page.

If the rating is 0 (no reported need associated with the topic over the past month), then go on to the next topic on the following page.

If the rating is 9 (not known or did not want to answer), then go on to the next topic on the following page.

Section 2

The purpose of Section 2 is to gain information about the level of support provided by friends and family during the past month. If the person interviewed has mentioned friends' names or relatives then personalise the question, but try not to exclude discussion of other people who might be helping; saying, for example, 'Does your mother, or any other relative,help you to keep clean and tidy? How about friends?' would personalise Section 2 of 'self-care'. Try to avoid commenting on the reported level of support, since this could be perceived as either critical or patronising. Do not ask how much help the person feels they need from friends and relatives.

Section 3

The purpose of Section 3 is to gain information about the current and required levels of support from local services over the past month. The two parts are best asked about separately. Try to personalise the questions by being specific about local services: for example, 'Do you talk to the nurses here when you feel sad? Anyone else here?' would be appropriate questions when interviewing a patient at a day centre. When rating, also consider the perceived effectiveness of an intervention: for example, when asking about psychotic symptoms, if the person is taking medication that is regularly reviewed, but reports that it does not relieve symptoms at all, then rate help received as 0.

The second part of Section 3 asks about people's perception of their need for help. Try to emphasise the word 'need' rather than asking how much help the person would 'like' from local services. Note that the question is not asking how much *extra* help is needed. Use the same rating scale as for the first question in this section. A rating of 0 indicates that the person perceives no need for help from local services. When the same rating is given for the two questions in Section 3, this indicates that the appropriate level of support is being provided by local services. When the rating is higher for the second question, this suggests the existence of unmet need.

Section 4

The purpose of Section 4 is to rate the person's perception of the appropriateness and effectiveness of interventions. It can be difficult to distinguish between the two questions in this section, but it could be that sometimes they are given different ratings. The first question asks about the appropriateness of current interventions – that is, does the person think *different* help should be given? The second asks about the person's satisfaction with the amount of help given – does the person think *more* help should be given? This section is intended to identify situations when the person feels either that the wrong type of help is being offered or that not enough of the right type of help is being offered.

Summary sheets

The summary sheets are designed for summarising the data collected using the CAN–EU (see Chapter 6). They are not exhaustive, and the use to which the data are put will dictate the best method of aggregation. Any aggregation of data will result in loss of information, so should be considered carefully.

The first sheet (p. 48) is a summary for a complete CAN–EU assessment. It also has a space for recording the total number of needs reported by the user and the staff member, and a row for recording the total for each column. When adding up these totals, always count a 9 (not known) as 0. As with all the summary sheets, completing these extra boxes involves analysis of the data collected during assessment. If all that is required is a record of the assessment, then the extra boxes do not have to be completed.

The totals in the 'need' column give an indication of the number of needs a person has (maximum 22) and how many are unmet (maximum score 44, if unmet needs exist in all 22 topics assessed). Comparison with previous summaries will show any changes over time. To find the number of needs, count how many 1s and 2s appear in the column. To find the total need, add up all the numbers in the column (remembering to count 9 as 0). The maximum possible total is 44. To make sense of the other totals (which again are found by adding the numbers in the respective columns) unfortunately requires some arithmetic, since the maximum possible total will vary according to how many needs are rated (since Sections 2–4 are only completed when a need exists). If required, the maximum possible score can be worked out using the method shown in each box: for example, the maximum possible total score for 'informal help given' rated by the user will be found by multiplying the number of needs rated by the user (NNU) by 3. Similarly, the number of needs rated by the staff (NNS) should go in the staff 'type of help' box. The worked examples will clarify what is required. The ratio of total rating over the maximum possible rating will indicate how much help is being received where needed, how much is needed, and what level of satisfaction exists.

We recommend that where possible the first summary sheet (page 48) be used, to allow easy comparison of staff and user views. However, the second and third sheets allow separate recording of staff and user assessments, and use the same calculations. The fourth sheet separates the topics assessed into groups, which may correspond to the interests of different mental health disciplines. For each subgroup the number of topics rated 1 or 2 is recorded (i.e. the number of needs within that subgroup), and the subtotal is found by adding up the numbers in the subgroup (as always, counting 9 as 0). This may inform the choice of the most appropriate professional to be appointed as the keyworker.

The summary sheets can be used as case-note entries.

5 Development and reliability of the CAN–EU

Paul McCrone, Morven Leese, Graham Thornicroft, Aart Schene, Helle Charlotte Knudsen, José Luis Vázquez-Barquero, Antonio Lasalvia, Sarah Padfield, Ian R. White, Gwyn Griffiths and the EPSILON Study Group

This section summarises the methods used in the EPSILON Study to establish the reliability of the European version of the Camberwell Assessment of Need (CAN–EU), presents the results, and discusses the implications of these findings. A more detailed account of the study is given in Chapters 1–3.

The assessment of individual patient outcomes increasingly takes into account the needs of those who suffer from mental illness. This emphasises the active role of the users of mental health services, and also raises a series of important questions. How can needs be defined, and by whom? How can they be measured and compared? What importance should be accorded to both met and unmet needs in the assessment of individual patients, and in the planning and evaluation of mental health services as a whole? How should the needs of people with schizophrenia be prioritised in relation to the needs of other diagnostic groups?

Development of the CAN–EU

The European version of the Camberwell Assessment of Need (CAN) was based on the CAN Research Version 3.0 (Phelan *et al*, 1995). This is an interviewer-administered instrument comprising 22 individual domains of need: accommodation, food, looking after the home, self-care, physical health, psychological distress, psychotic symptoms, information about condition and treatment, daytime activities, company, safety to self, safety to others, alcohol, drugs, intimate relationships, sexual expression, basic education, child care, transport, using a telephone, money and welfare benefits. There is good agreement between staff and user ratings of the overall numbers of needs, although there may be substantial differences for individual items. It is important to note that in the EPSILON Study the service user (patient) ratings were used.

Each item of the CAN–EU contains the same question structure. The first question asks whether a need exists, and if it does, whether it is a met or an unmet need. If there is no need in any particular area, then the interviewer proceeds straight to the next item. If a met or unmet need does exist, then further questions relating to service receipt for that item are asked. The first of these finds out how much care is received from friends or relatives (0, no help; 1, low help; 2, moderate help; 3, high help). The same question is asked about care received from formal services and also how much care is required from formal services. Finally, the person being interviewed is asked whether overall they receive the right sort of help, and whether they receive the right amount of help. Both of these are rated as 0 (no) or 1 (yes).

Summary scores of the total number of needs (the number of 1s or 2s), the met needs (the number of 1s) and the unmet needs (the number of 2s) are computed. If the number of valid items (i.e. excluding missing values) needs is 18 or more, a pro-rated total is computed from the valid items, otherwise the summary score is regarded as missing.

The EPSILON Study

The Camberwell Assessment of Need was one of the five mental health research instruments chosen by the EPSILON Study to be produced in standardised versions in five European languages – Danish, Dutch, English, Italian and Spanish (see Chapter 1). This involved a rigorous conversion process of accurate and independent translation and back-translation from the original language into the other four languages, checks of cross-cultural applicability using focus groups (see Chapter 2), and assessment of instrument reliability. Although it is now relatively common for the authors of outcome scales to publish details of scale reliability in the original language, it is rare for the authors of translated versions to repeat the reliability exercise in the new languages or indeed to do more than undertake a literal translation. The EPSILON Study was therefore designed to undertake this procedure for each of the five scales into all the study languages in a comprehensive and scientifically rigorous manner.

Study sites

Six partners in five centres joined forces for this collaborative study, with the teams located in Amsterdam, Copenhagen, London (Centre for the Economics of Mental Health and Section of Community Psychiatry, Institute of Psychiatry), Santander and Verona (see Chapter 1 for details).

Participants

Participants in the study were adults aged 18–65 years, selected as representative of all people suffering from schizophrenia utilising mental health services in each of the five study sites. Study samples were identified either from psychiatric case registers (in Copenhagen and Verona) or case-loads of local special mental health services (in-patient, out-patient and community). Patients included had been in contact with mental health services during the 3 months before the start of the study in 1997. Only patients with an ICD–10 research diagnosis of schizophrenia (code F20) were finally included. The screening procedure and exclusion criteria are detailed in Chapter 1.

Translation

The study included the conversion of each of the five scales from their original language into the other four study languages. The procedures of translation, back-translation and assessment by focus groups are described in Chapter 2.

Interviewing and data preparation

All interviewers received training at the Institute of Psychiatry, London, UK, in the use of the study instruments. There were regular contacts to ensure standard use of instruments and a series of study co-ordinating meetings. Data consistency and homogeneity were ensured by the coordinating centre (in London) preparing the Statistical Package for the Social Sciences (SPSS) templates used at all the participating sites. Consistent data structures were adhered to.

Reliability assessment

Reliability testing was conducted on several levels depending on the nature of the responses involved and whether the instruments are administered as interviews or questionnaires. The methodology is discussed in detail in Chapter 3. Three kinds of reliability test were used: (a) Cronbach's α statistic, to estimate the internal consistency of scales and sub-scales consisting of more than one item; (b) Cohen's κ statistic to estimate the interrater reliability and test–retest reliability of single items where these are expressed as binary variables; and (c) intraclass correlations, to estimate the interrater reliability and test–retest reliability of scales and sub-scales. These statistics are discussed in Streiner & Norman (1995). Each step in the analysis was described in an analysis protocol, which was followed by all sites.

First, summary statistics were computed for each site, and differences in sample variances were explored using the Levene test (Levene, 1960). Cronbach's α was computed for each site, and for the pooled sample, and a test for differences in α values between sites was performed (Feldt et al, 1987). Intraclass correlation coefficients (ICCs) were computed by maximum likelihood estimation of a variance components model, with patients entered as random effects, and (in the case of pooled estimates) site entered as a fixed effect. The data for each patient were either all time 1 ratings (for interrater reliability), or all ratings by the first rater (for test–retest reliability). All available data were used for these analyses, including cases where only one rating was present; however, values of n quoted in the tables relating to reliability are the numbers of complete pairs. Only at one site (Verona) were there sufficient raters to estimate a specific interrater component of variance. However, for consistency in estimation between the sites, rater was not specifically included in the model. Interrater variance is thus reflected in the ICC by being incorporated in the error variance.

The ratio of the between-patient component of variance to total variance was used to estimate the ICC, and the delta technique (Dunn, 1989) was used to obtain standard errors for the ICC from the variance–covariance matrix for the components. Fisher's Z transformation was applied (Donner & Bull, 1983), and differences between sites were then tested for significance by the method of weighting (Armitage & Berry, 1994), before transforming back to the ICC scale. The standard error of measurement was obtained from the 'error' component of variance. Pooled reliability of the individual items was estimated, without between-site testing. Finally, a paired t-test on the test–retest data was carried out in order to assess systematic changes from time 1 to time 2.

For reasons of comparability, all sites used the same procedure and the same software for all instruments: SPSS 7.5 or higher, the Amsterdam α-testing program ALPHA.EXE based on Feldt et al (1987), and Excel for tests of the homogeneity of ICCs. Test–retest reliability was conducted at intervals of 1–2 weeks, although in a few cases up to 7 weeks elapsed, depending on the practicalities of contacting patients. The same rater interviewed at test and retest. For the CAN, patients' responses are rated by an interviewer, and therefore interrater reliability is an issue as well as test–retest. For interrater reliability, a second rater present at the interviews rated in parallel with the primary interviewer who asked the questions of the patient. The numbers of raters at time 1 and time 2 were as follows: Amsterdam: 4, 4; Copenhagen: 5, 5; London: 2, 5; Santander: 3, 3; Verona: 11, 13.

Answers to the service receipt part of the CAN–EU domains depend on the answers to the first part (presence of a need), and therefore interrater reliability for the subsequent sections is hard to define, since the parallel rater has no control over the flow of questions. Furthermore, the service receipt sections are mainly useful in a clinical situation. For these reasons, and in common with reliability testing of the original CAN, these sections have not been analysed here for reliability purposes.

Table 5.1 The Camberwell Assessment of Need – European Version (CAN–EU): total, met and unmet needs in the pooled sample and by site; results of primary rater at time 1

	Pooled n=400		Amsterdam n=59		Copenhagen n=51		London n=84		Santander n=100		Verona n=106		Test of equality of means (P)	Test of equality of s.d.[1] (P)
	mean	s.d.	mean	s.d.	mean	s.d.	mean	s.d.	mean	s.d.	mean	s.d.		
Total needs	5.35	3.07	6.31	2.96	5.19	3.39	5.95	2.78	4.81	2.52	4.93	3.28	<0.01	0.02
Met needs	3.56	2.26	3.79	2.38	3.86	2.46	3.77	1.88	3.19	1.64	3.46	2.80	0.27	<0.01
Unmet needs	1.79	1.98	2.52	2.02	1.33	1.96	2.18	2.09	1.61	1.68	1.48	2.00	<0.01	0.42

1. Levine test.

Results

Table 5.1 gives the summary statistics for the primary rater at time 1, including the results of a homogeneity of variance test. Mean total needs and unmet needs differed significantly between sites, with Amsterdam and London tending to show higher values than the other three sites on both measures. Of more relevance to the reliability estimation is the lack of homogeneity in variance for met and total needs, as shown by the Levene test in Table 5.1.

The α coefficients, which reflect correlations between individual CAN items, were moderate to low (Table 5.2). For total needs, the pooled α was 0.64 (95% CI 0.58–0.70). Only for met needs (pooled mean 0.48, 95% CI 0.40–0.56) was there strong evidence for differences between sites, with Santander having the lowest value at 0.16. For unmet needs (pooled mean 0.58, 95% CI 0.51–0.64) the differences were less marked, but Copenhagen showed a somewhat higher value than the other sites, at 0.70.

The ICCs between the two time points are given in Table 5.3, which shows that test–retest reliability is at an acceptable level. There was no significant difference between sites, except for unmet needs. Pooled values were 0.85 (95% CI 0.82–0.88) for total needs, 0.69 (95% CI 0.63–0.74) for met needs and 0.78 (95% CI 0.74–0.82) for unmet needs.

For estimating κ coefficients for the individual items, unmet, met and total needs were each expressed as binary variables in turn. Table 5.4 shows that κ coefficients for test–retest reliability were high for total needs (0.55–0.84), and moderately high for met needs (0.40–0.76, excluding κ for met needs for drugs, which was zero) and unmet needs (0.34–0.85). Standard errors for these κ estimates were typically 0.06, 0.08 and 0.09, respectively. Only one item had a κ coefficient below 0.4 (unmet needs for physical health).

There was evidence of site differences in interrater reliability (Table 5.5) for total, met and unmet needs. However, all the sites had coefficients for total and met needs above 0.8. In the case of unmet

Table 5.2 Internal consistency of the Camberwell Assessment of Need – European Version (CAN–EU): α coefficients[1] (95% CI) in the pooled sample and by site

	Pooled n=327	Amsterdam n=57	Copenhagen n=42	London n=69	Santander n=94	Verona n=65	Test of equality of α (P)
Total needs	0.64(0.58–0.70)	0.64(0.49–0.76)	0.73(0.59–0.83)	0.55(0.39–0.69)	0.61(0.48–0.71)	0.67(0.54–0.77)	0.42
Met needs	0.48(0.40–0.56)	0.58(0.41–0.72)	0.54(0.37–0.72)	0.36(0.11–0.56)	0.16(−0.10–0.39)	0.62(0.47–0.74)	0.03
Unmet needs	0.58(0.51–0.64)	0.52(0.32–0.68)	0.70(0.56–0.82)	0.55(0.38–0.69)	0.57(0.43–0.72)	0.58(0.42–0.72)	0.04

1. α estimated only for cases with completed data (22 items).

Table 5.3 Test–retest reliability of the Camberwell Assessment of Need – European Version (CAN–EU) summary scores in the pooled sample and by site

	Pooled $n=198^2$		Amsterdam $n=51$		Copenhagen $n=16$		London $n=46$		Santander $n=48$		Verona $n=37$		Test of equality of ICCs
	ICC	(s.e.)$_m$	ICC	(s.e.)$_m$	ICC	(s.e.)$_m$	ICC	(s.e.)$_m$	ICC	(s.e.)$_m$	ICC	(s.e.)$_m$	P
Total needs	0.85	1.12	0.81	1.23	0.90	1.02	0.82	1.13	0.89	0.82	0.85	1.26	0.33
Met needs	0.69	1.22	0.65	1.35	0.75	1.15	0.71	1.01	0.75	0.81	0.65	1.59	0.70
Unmet needs	0.78	0.90	0.72	1.08	0.84	0.84	0.86	0.76	0.83	0.69	0.69	1.06	0.03

ICC, intraclass correlation coefficient; (s.e.)$_m$, standard error of measurement (square root of error components of variance).

needs, coefficients for Amsterdam, Santander and Verona were under 0.8, although they were all still over 0.65. The pooled estimates were 0.93 (95% CI 0.92–0.95) for total needs, 0.85 (95% CI 0.81–0.87) for met needs and 0.79 (95% CI 0.75–0.83) for unmet needs.

Interrater reliability for individual items, pooled over sites (Table 5.6) was very good for total needs (0.75–0.99) and met needs (0.57–0.95), and moderately good for unmet needs (0.41–0.83). Standard errors were typically 0.04, 0.07 and 0.10, respectively. All items had κ coefficients over 0.4.

Paired sample t-tests revealed a tendency for a decrease in the rating of total needs over time, pooled across sites, but this was significant only at a borderline level (P=0.053). At individual sites, there were no significant differences between mean scores at test and retest, with the exception of

Table 5.4 Test–retest reliability of the Camberwell Assessment of Need – European Version (CAN–EU) items in the pooled sample

CAN no.	Area of need	Agreement (%)	Total needs	Met needs	Unmet needs
1	Accommodation	92	0.84	0.76	0.60
2	Food	91	0.82	0.74	0.77
3	Looking after the home	85	0.66	0.60	0.75
4	Self-care	92	0.74	0.62	0.62
5	Daytime activities	82	0.74	0.60	0.73
6	Physical health	84	0.70	0.66	**0.34**
7	Psychotic symptoms	86	0.75	0.66	0.70
8	Information about condition and treatment	80	0.69	**0.49**	**0.50**
9	Psychological distress	72	0.64	**0.43**	**0.55**
10	Safety to self	93	0.76	**0.57**	0.68
11	Safety to others	95	0.60	**0.51**	**0.45**
12	Alcohol	96	0.75	0.70	0.62
13	Drugs	97	0.65	$-^1$	0.85
14	Company	73	**0.59**	**0.44**	**0.53**
15	Intimate relationships	82	**0.55**	**0.54**	**0.51**
16	Sexual expression	88	**0.59**	**0.40**	**0.58**
17	Child care	97	0.76	0.61	0.79
18	Basic education	92	0.70	0.67	**0.54**
19	Using a telephone	98	0.84	**0.59**	0.74
20	Transport	93	0.79	0.72	0.78
21	Money	86	0.74	0.60	0.62
22	Welfare benefits	91	0.68	**0.53**	0.72

Percentage agreement over all three needs and κ coefficients; κ<0.6 in **bold** type.
1. Low base rate (4 and 6 cases of met need at times 1 and 2, respectively) with no agreement.

Table 5.5 Interrater reliability of the Camberwell Assessment of Need – European Version (CAN–EU) in the pooled sample and by site

	Pooled $n=274$		Amsterdam $n=47$		Copenhagen $n=40$		London $n=79$		Santander $n=50$		Verona $n=58$		Test of equality of ICCs
	ICC	(s.e.)$_m$	ICC	(s.e.)$_m$	ICC	(s.e.)$_m$	ICC	(s.e.)$_m$	ICC	(s.e.)$_m$	ICC	(s.e.)$_m$	P
Total needs	0.93	0.77	0.90	0.91	0.93	0.84	0.99	0.29	0.93	0.65	0.91	0.93	<0.01
Met needs	0.85	0.86	0.83	0.95	0.82	0.99	0.96	0.38	0.82	0.72	0.83	1.08	<0.01
Unmet needs	0.79	0.85	0.71	1.01	0.84	0.75	0.98	0.33	0.77	0.77	0.68	1.06	<0.01

ICC, intraclass correlation coefficient; (s.e.)$_m$, standard error of measurement (square root of error components of variance).

total needs in Verona, where the time 2 total values were rated lower: 4.39 at time 2 compared with 5.11 at time 1, difference 0.72 (95% CI 0.52–0.92), $P=0.001$. This is could be a chance finding, given the large number of tests employed.

Discussion

The assessment of the reliability of the CAN–EU did not include a specific test of face validity. However, focus groups were used in the translation process, and these indicated that the CAN–EU was largely acceptable in its format and content. This confirmed the attainment of face validity for the original English version (Phelan *et al*, 1995). Very high internal consistency between the items for the CAN–EU is not expected or even necessarily desirable, and the moderate levels of α are quite acceptable in this context. Indeed, they are not surprising, given the diverse range of needs assessed with the instrument, which were deliberately selected to cover the entire range of difficulties commonly encountered by people suffering from severe mental illnesses. In this context the α coefficients are not that informative, but have been reported here for completeness.

The low value for α for met needs for Santander is interesting, and may be connected with the lower level and smaller degree of variation in met needs at that particular site, as shown in Table 5.1. Alternatively, it may be connected with one particular item, 'help with psychotic symptoms'. When this item is removed, the α is doubled to 0.32, more in keeping with its value at other sites.

Overall, the test–retest reliability is at least moderately good, although usually lower than interrater reliability. Lack of reliability may, in some cases, be due to changes in patient status that occurred between the two time points, in addition to lack of consistency in a patient's responses from one time point to the next. However, interviews were generally made within intervals of 1–2 weeks, so real changes in status were unlikely.

Interrater reliability is excellent, with only a slight fall-off for unmet needs. Although there were significant differences between sites, all values of interrater reliability coefficients were over 0.65. The two slightly lower reliabilities for unmet needs (Amsterdam and Verona) are due to higher standard errors of measurement rather than the differences in variances between the samples shown in Table 5.1. It should be noted that Verona had a larger pool of primary raters and, in this respect, the data from that site may more realistically reflect the range of raters who might use the instrument in practice. The very small standard error of measurement in London might reflect a longer history of CAN training and use.

For individual items, both for test–retest and interrater reliability, the items with the lowest κ values tend to be those having low base rates for the need: for example, drugs. Two items showed both low κ and low percentage agreement in the test–retest comparison: 'psychological distress' (item 9) and 'company' (item 14). These two items are not of this character, and there seems to be no

Table 5.6 Interrater reliability of the Camberwell Assessment of Need – European Version (CAN–EU) items in the pooled sample

CAN no.	Area of need	Agreement (%)	Total needs	Met needs	Unmet needs
1	Accommodation	95	0.94	0.83	**0.41**
2	Food	95	0.88	0.86	0.72
3	Looking after the home	94	0.86	0.84	0.76
4	Self-care	98	0.95	0.94	0.66
5	Daytime activities	90	0.93	0.79	0.73
6	Physical health	95	0.92	0.90	0.73
7	Psychotic symptoms	86	0.83	0.66	0.64
8	Information about condition and treatment	87	0.92	0.69	**0.45**
9	Psychological distress	89	0.94	0.78	0.73
10	Safety to self	96	0.82	0.75	0.83
11	Safety to others	99	0.84	0.95	0.83
12	Alcohol	99	0.89	0.92	0.75
13	Drugs	98	0.94	**0.57**	0.80
14	Company	88	0.97	0.74	0.77
15	Intimate relationships	92	0.94	0.77	0.78
16	Sexual expression	91	0.84	0.72	**0.57**
17	Child care	96	0.79	0.61	0.69
18	Basic education	97	0.84	0.88	0.71
19	Using a telephone	98	0.75	0.83	0.66
20	Transport	98	0.99	0.90	0.83
21	Money	93	0.91	0.87	0.68
22	Welfare benefits	94	0.86	0.68	0.74

Percentage agreement over all three needs and κ coefficients; κ<0.6 in **bold** type.

obvious pattern in the inconsistent responses over time. It may be that these two items are hard to rate because they are very much related to mood and reflect relatively transient situations.

A point that applies generally, both over time and also between raters, is that there are greater levels of agreement for total needs than for the component items. However, the very skewed nature of the data relating to individual items (i.e. the low base rates in many cases) makes reliability tests problematic. Indeed, it reduces the feasibility of analysing these variables individually, except in very large samples.

Mean scores did not differ significantly between test and retest, except for one score in one site. The pooled ratings for total needs did decrease slightly over time (at a borderline level of significance), but in general there is little evidence of substantial increase or decrease over time, a problem that might occur if patients tended to reflect on and modify their ideas following an interview. In these respects the CAN–EU can be seen to be stable over time.

This analysis has concentrated on the three total needs scores, rather than individual items. This is because the 22 CAN–EU items, although clearly important in considering the needs of individual patients, are of limited use for analytical purposes when treated in isolation, since most of them are encountered infrequently in individual cases. Similarly, the sections of the CAN–EU relating to levels of formal and informal care received, and formal care required, are more relevant to clinical use rather than research. With large samples, the data on particular needs and on care required or received could be analysed, but such samples have hitherto been scarce.

Bearing in mind these caveats, we suggest that the summary scores for the CAN–EU (total, met and unmet needs) are generally reliable over time and between raters. Despite some evidence for differences in levels of reliability between sites for unmet needs at test–retest comparisons, and between raters for all three total scores, the results are good at each site, and encouraging for the use of this instrument in its five translations.

References and further reading

American Psychiatric Association (1987) *Diagnostic and Statistical Manual of Mental Disorders* (3rd edn, revised) (DSM–III–R). Washington, DC: APA.

Armitage, P. & Berry, G. (1994) *Statistical Methods in Medical Research* (3rd edn). Oxford: Blackwell Scientific.

Beecham, J. & Knapp, M. (1992) Costing psychiatric interventions. In *Measuring Mental Health Needs* (eds G. Thornicroft, C. R. Brewin & J. Wing), pp. 200–224. London: Gaskell.

Donner, A. & Bull, S. (1983) Inferences concerning a common intraclass correlation coefficient. *Biometrics*, **39**, 771–775.

Dunn, G. (1989) *Design and Analysis of Reliability Studies*. London: Edward Arnold.

Feldt, L. S., Woodruff, D. J. & Salih, F. A. (1987) Statistical inference for coefficient alpha. *Applied Psychological Measurement*, **11**, 93–103.

Johnson, S., Salvador-Carulla, L. & the EPCAT group (1998) Description and classification of mental health services: a European perspective. *European Psychiatry*, **13**, 333–341.

Levene, H. (1960) Tests for equality of variances. In *Contributions to Probability and Statistics: Essays in Honor of Harold Hotelling* (eds I. Olkin, S. G. Ghurye, W. Hoeffding, *et al*), pp. 278–292. Stanford, CA: Stanford University Press.

Overall, J. & Gorham, D. (1962) Brief Psychiatric Rating Scale. *Psychological Reports*, **10**, 799–812.

Phelan, M., Slade, M., Thornicroft, G., *et al* (1995) The Camberwell Assessment of Need: the validity and reliability of an instrument to assess the needs of people with severe mental illness. *British Journal of Psychiatry*, **167**, 589–595.

Streiner, D. & Norman, G. (1995) *Health Measurement Scales: A Practical Guide to their Development and Use*. Oxford: Oxford University Press.

World Health Organization (1992) *Schedules for Clinical Assessment in Neuropsychiatry* (ed.-in-chief J. K. Wing). Geneva: WHO.

6 Camberwell Assessment of Need – European Version

Paul McCrone, Mike Slade, Morven Leese,
Graham Thornicroft and the EPSILON Study Group

CAN–EU
Complete assessment summary sheet

User name _____ Date of assessment ____/____/____

Staff name _____ Date of assessment ____/___/____

	Need		Informal help given		Formal help given		Formal help needed		Type of help		Amount of help
Rating	0,1,2,9		0,1,2,3,9		0,1,2,3,9		0,1,2,3,9		0,1,9		0,1,9
User/Staff rating	1U	1S	2U	2S	3U	3S	4U	4S	5U	5S	6U
1 Accommodation											
2 Food											
3 Looking after home											
4 Self-care											
5 Daytime activities											
6 Physical health											
7 Psychotic symptoms											
8 Information											
9 Psychological distress											
10 Safety to self											
11 Safety to others											
12 Alcohol											
13 Drugs											
14 Company											
15 Intimate relationships											
16 Sexual expression											
17 Child care											
18 Education											
19 Telephone											
20 Transport											
21 Money											
22 Benefits											
Number of met needs (Number of 1s)			/////	/////	/////	/////	/////	/////	/////	/////	/////
Number of unmet needs (Number of 2s)			/////	/////	/////	/////	/////	/////	/////	/////	/////
Total number of needs (Number of 1s and 2s)			/////	/////	/////	/////	/////	/////	/////	/////	/////
Total level of help given & needed, & satisfaction (Add scores, rate 9 as 0)	/////	/////									

CAN–EU
User assessment summary sheet

User name _____ Date of assessment ____/____/____

Interviewer _____

	Need	Informal help given	Formal help given	Formal help needed	Type of help	Amount of help
Rating	0,1,2,9	0,1,2,3,9	0,1,2,3,9	0,1,2,3,9	0,1,9	0,1,9
User/Staff rating	1U	2U	3U	4U	5U	6U
1 Accommodation						
2 Food						
3 Looking after home						
4 Self-care						
5 Daytime activities						
6 Physical health						
7 Psychotic symptoms						
8 Information						
9 Psychological distress						
10 Safety to self						
11 Safety to others						
12 Alcohol						
13 Drugs						
14 Company						
15 Intimate relationships						
16 Sexual expression						
17 Child care						
18 Education						
19 Telephone						
20 Transport						
21 Money						
22 Benefits						
Number of met needs (Number of 1s)		/////	/////	/////	/////	/////
Number of unmet needs (Number of 2s)		/////	/////	/////	/////	/////
Total number of needs (Number of 1s and 2s)		/////	/////	/////	/////	/////
Total level of help given & needed, & satisfaction (Add scores, rate 9 as 0)	/////					

CAN–EU
Staff assessment summary sheet

User name _____

Staff name _____ Date of assessment ____/____/____

	Need	Informal help given	Formal help given	Formal help needed	Type of help
Rating	0,1,2,9	0,1,2,3,9	0,1,2,3,9	0,1,2,3,9	0,1,9
User/Staff rating	1S	2S	3S	4S	5S
1 Accommodation					
2 Food					
3 Looking after home					
4 Self-care					
5 Daytime activities					
6 Physical health					
7 Psychotic symptoms					
8 Information					
9 Psychological distress					
10 Safety to self					
11 Safety to others					
12 Alcohol					
13 Drugs					
14 Company					
15 Intimate relationships					
16 Sexual expression					
17 Child care					
18 Education					
19 Telephone					
20 Transport					
21 Money					
22 Benefits					
Number of met needs (Number of 1s)					
Number of unmet needs (Number of 2s)					
Total number of needs (Number of 1s and 2s)					
Total level of help given & needed, & satisfaction (Add scores, rate 9 as 0)					

CAN–EU   Grouped assessment summary sheet

Client name / ID _____ Date ____ /____/ ____

Staff name / ID _____ Date ____ /____/ ____

	Need		Informal help given		Formal help needed		Formal help		Type of help		Amount of help
Rating (9=not known)	0, 1 or 2		0, 1, 2 or 3		0, 1, 2 or 3		0, 1, 2 or 3		0 or 1		0 or 1
CAN box number	01	02	03	04	05	06	07	08	09	10	11
User/Staff rating	U	S	U	S	U	S	U	S	U	S	U
Basic											
1 Accommodation											
2 Food											
5 Daytime activities											
No. of 1s and 2s (max 3)											
Sub-total (max 6)											
Health											
6 Physical health											
7 Psychotic symptoms											
9 Psychological distress											
10 Safety to self											
11 Safety to others											
12 Alcohol											
13 Drugs											
No. of 1s and 2s (max 7)											
Sub-total (max 14)											
Social											
14 Company											
15 Intimate relationships											
16 Sexual expression											
No. of 1s and 2s (max 3)											
Sub-total (max 6)											
Functioning											
3 Looking after the home											
4 Self-care											
17 Child care											
18 Education											
21 Money											
No. of 1s and 2s (max 5)											
Sub-total (max 10)											
Services											
8 Information											
19 Telephone											
20 Transport											
22 Benefits											
No. of 1s and 2s (max 4)											
Sub-total (max 8)											

CAN–EU Worked example

A worked example of the four summary sheets is now given, based on (fictitious) interviews with Chris, a mental health service user, and her keyworker Richard.

Interview with Chris

Chris enjoys living in her hostel, although she would like to have her own accommodation, and says the keyworker refuses to refer her. She occasionally gets 'moaned at' by hostel staff to clean her bedroom, but would like some practical help from them. She does not need any help in keeping herself clean. Every day, she attends a day centre where she has a meal. All other meals are supplied at the hostel and she needs this level of help. Chris reports that the centre is boring, and makes her feelings of loneliness even worse. She does not know what she would prefer to do during the day, but is unhappy with the current arrangements. The staff have been very helpful already in arranging for her to attend, but she feels she would need a lot of help with finding more enjoyable things to do. She is often lonely or feels low, and rings her mother every month or so about this. Apart from that, she gets no help with her difficulties from friends or relatives. She would like to talk to Richard about how she feels when she is lonely or down, but does not get the chance at present. She is physically well, and although there is nothing wrong with her thoughts or nerves, they make her have an injection. She has never felt like hitting anyone else or harming herself, and does not drink or take drugs. Chris reports that she is single and has no sex life, both of which are 'okay'. She has no children. Her reading is not so good and she would like Richard to fill in forms for her, although he does not help in this way at present. Chris has to ask before she can use the pay-phone in the hostel. Although the hostel staff always let her use the telephone, she would prefer her own telephone in her room. She has a bus pass, which is 'wonderful'. She has no difficulty budgeting, and Richard is sorting out a new benefit for her.

Interview with Richard, Chris's keyworker

Chris lives in a hostel for people with mental health problems, which is the right sort of accommodation for her. All meals are provided for her by the hostel and day centre, which is needed. Hostel staff occasionally help tidy her bedroom (which Chris needs), but she keeps herself clean. She attends a day centre most days, and would be lonely if not attending. Chris has been quite happy in the past month. Physically she is well. She has been diagnosed as having a psychotic illness, which is reviewed by her psychiatrist every 3 months. Richard would like to give Chris a comprehensive education about her illness, but whenever he tries to talk to her about this she says she does not want to hear anything about it. However, sometimes Chris says that her mother told her she is not ill, so Richard is not sure if Chris discusses her mental health with her mother. Apart from this, Richard believes that she has no friends or contact with family. She is not suicidal or violent, and does not drink or take drugs. Richard believes (but is not sure) that Chris does not want a relationship with anyone at the moment, and has never asked if Chris has any sexual problems. Chris has no children. Since Chris cannot read, either Richard or the hostel staff fill in any forms for her. Richard is not sure that this is the most appropriate help with literacy, but is unsure what else could be done. She has a bus pass and access to a telephone at the hostel when she asks, which meets her needs in these areas. She finds it hard to save money, but 'gets by'. Richard has recently applied on her behalf for the Disability Living Allowance.

CAN–EU
Example of completed assessment summary sheet

| User name | Chris | Date of assessment | 10 / 11 / 03 |
| Staff name | Richard | Date of assessment | 10 / 11 / 03 |

	Need		Informal help given		Formal help given		Formal help needed		Type of help		Amount of help
Rating	0,1,2,9		0,1,2,3,9		0,1,2,3,9		0,1,2,3,9		0,1,9		0,1,9
User/Staff rating	1U	1S	2U	2S	3U	3S	4U	4S	5U	5S	6U
1 Accommodation	1	1	0	0	3	3	2	3	0	1	1
2 Food	1	1	0	0	3	3	3	3	1	1	1
3 Looking after home	1	1	0	0	1	2	2	2	0	1	0
4 Self-care	0	0									
5 Daytime activities	2	1	0	0	0	3	3	3	0	1	1
6 Physical health	0	0									
7 Psychotic symptoms	0	1		9		1		1		1	
8 Information	0	2		9		0		3		1	
9 Psychological distress	1	0	1		0		1		0		0
10 Safety to self	0	0									
11 Safety to others	0	0									
12 Alcohol	0	0									
13 Drugs	0	0									
14 Company	2	1	1	9	0	3	1	3	0	1	0
15 Intimate relationships	0	0									
16 Sexual expression	0	9									
17 Child care	0	0									
18 Education	2	1	0	0	0	1	1	9	0	9	0
19 Telephone	1	1	0	0	1	1	3	1	0	1	1
20 Transport	1	1	0	0	1	1	1	1	1	1	1
21 Money	0	0									
22 Benefits	1	1	0	0	2	2	2	2	1	1	1
Number of met needs (Number of 1s)	7	10									
Number of unmet needs (Number of 2s)	3	1									
Total number of needs (Number of 1s and 2s)	10	11									
Total level of help given & needed, & satisfaction (Add scores, rate 9 as 0)			2	0	11	20	19	22	3	10	6

CAN–EU
Example of completed user assessment summary sheet

User name ___Chris___   Date of assessment ___10___ / ___11___ / ___03___

Interviewer _____

	Need	Informal help given	Formal help given	Formal help needed	Type of help	Amount of help
Rating	0,1,2,9	0,1,2,3,9	0,1,2,3,9	0,1,2,3,9	0,1,9	0,1,9
User/Staff rating	1U	2U	3U	4U	5U	6U
1 Accommodation	1	0	3	2	0	1
2 Food	1	0	3	3	1	1
3 Looking after home	1	0	1	2	0	0
4 Self-care	0					
5 Daytime activities	2	0	0	3	0	1
6 Physical health	0					
7 Psychotic symptoms	0					
8 Information	0					
9 Psychological distress	1	1	0	1	0	0
10 Safety to self	0					
11 Safety to others	0					
12 Alcohol	0					
13 Drugs	0					
14 Company	2	1	0	1	0	0
15 Intimate relationships	0					
16 Sexual expression	0					
17 Child care	0					
18 Education	2	0	0	1	0	0
19 Telephone	1	0	1	3	0	0
20 Transport	1	0	1	1	1	1
21 Money	0					
22 Benefits	1	0	2	2	1	1
Number of met needs (Number of 1s)	7					
Number of unmet needs (Number of 2s)	3					
Total number of needs (Number of 1s and 2s)	10					
Total level of help given & needed, & satisfaction (Add scores, rate 9 as 0)		2	11	19	3	5

CAN–EU
Example of completed staff assessment summary sheet

User name ___Chris___

Staff name ___Richard___ Date of assessment ___11___ / ___11___ / ___94___

	Need	Informal help given	Formal help given	Formal help needed	Type of help
Rating	0,1,2,9	0,1,2,3,9	0,1,2,3,9	0,1,2,3,9	0,1,9
User/Staff rating	1S	2S	3S	4S	5S
1 Accommodation	1	0	3	3	1
2 Food	1	0	3	3	1
3 Looking after home	1	0	2	2	1
4 Self-care	0				
5 Daytime activities	1	0	3	3	1
6 Physical health	0				
7 Psychotic symptoms	1	9	1	1	1
8 Information	2	9	0	3	1
9 Psychological distress	0				
10 Safety to self	0				
11 Safety to others	0				
12 Alcohol	0				
13 Drugs	0				
14 Company	1	9	3	3	1
15 Intimate relationships	9				
16 Sexual expression	0				
17 Child care	0				
18 Education	1	0	1	9	9
19 Telephone	1	0	1	1	1
20 Transport	1	0	1	1	1
21 Money	0				
22 Benefits	1	0	2	2	1
Number of met needs (Number of 1s)	10				
Number of unmet needs (Number of 2s)	1				
Total number of needs (Number of 1s and 2s)	11				
Total level of help given & needed, & satisfaction (Add scores, rate 9 as 0)		0	20	22	10

CAN–EU　Example of completed grouped assessment summary sheet

Client name / ID　Chris　　　　　　　　　　Date　10 / 11 / 94
Staff name / ID　Richard　　　　　　　　　Date　11 / 11 / 94

	Need		Informal help given		Formal help needed		Formal help		Type of help		Amount of help
Rating (9=not known)	0, 1 or 2		0, 1, 2 or 3		0, 1, 2 or 3		0, 1, 2 or 3		0 or 1		0 or 1
CAN box number	01	02	03	04	05	06	07	08	09	10	11
User / staff rating	U	S	U	S	U	S	U	S	U	S	U
Basic											
1　Accommodation	1	1	0	0	3	3	2	3	0	1	1
2　Food	1	1	0	0	0	3	3	3	1	1	1
5　Daytime activities	2	1	0	0	0	3	3	3	0	1	1
No. of 1s and 2s (max 3)	3	3									
Sub-total (max 6)	4	3									
Health											
6　Physical health	0	0									
7　Psychotic symptoms	0	1		9		1		1		1	1
9　Psychological distress	1	0	1		0		1		0		0
10　Safety to self	0	0									
11　Safety to others	0	0									
12　Alcohol	0	0									
13　Drugs	0	0									
No. of 1s and 2s (max 7)	1	1									
Sub-total (max 14)	1	1									
Social											
14　Company	2	1	1	9	0	3	1	3	0	1	0
15　Intimate relationships	0	0									
16　Sexual expression	0	9									
No. of 1s and 2s (max 3)	1	1									
Sub-total (max 6)	2	1									
Functioning											
3　Looking after the home	1	1	0	0	1	2	2	2	0	1	0
4　Self-care	0	0									
17　Child care	0	0									
18　Education	2	1	0	0	0	1	1	9	0	9	0
21　Money	0	0									
No. of 1s and 2s (max 5)	2	2									
Sub-total (max 10)	3	2									
Services											
8　Information	0	2		9		0		3		1	
19　Telephone	1	0	0		1		3		0		0
20　Transport	1	1	0	0	1	1	1	1	1	1	1
22　Benefits	1	1	0	0	2	2	2	2	1	1	1
No. of 1s and 2s (max 4)	3	3									
Sub-total (max 8)	3	4									

Publishing results from the CAN–EU

When publishing CAN–EU data, the following two tables can be used. Please acknowledge them as coming from:

> Slade, M., Thornicroft, G., Loftus, L., *et al* (1999) *Camberwell Assessment of Need (CAN).* London: Gaskell.

It is suggested that the data be presented separately for staff and user assessments. The amount of help data are only included for the user tables. The first table gives information about the overall level of need and help in the sample population:

Suggested table to present summarised results of CAN–EU

Mean number of needs Maximum: 22	
Mean need rating 22 topics, each scoring 1 for a partially met need or 2 for an unmet need Maximum: 44	
Mean level of informal help given where need exists Rating: 0 (none) – 3 (high) Maximum: 3	
Mean level of formal help given, where need exists Rating: 0 (none) – 3 (high) Maximum: 3	
Mean level of formal help needed, where need exists Rating: 0 (none) – 3 (high) Maximum: 3	
Mean satisfaction with type of help, where need exists Rating: 0 (none) – 1 (satisfied) Maximum: 1	
Mean satisfaction with amount of help where need exists Rating: 0 (not satisfied) – 1 (satisfied) Maximum: 1	

Suggested table to present summarised data about individual needs domains

	Number with met or unmet need n (%)	Number with unmet need n (%)	Mean level of informal help given, where need exists 0=none 3=high	Mean level of formal help given, where need exists 0=none 3=high	Mean level of formal help needed, where need exists 0=none 3=high	Mean satisfaction with type of help, where need exists 0=not satisfied 1=satisfied	Mean satisfaction with amount of help, where need exists 0=not satisfied 1=satisfied
1 Accommodation							
2 Food							
3 Looking after home							
4 Self-care							
5 Daytime activities							
6 Physical health							
7 Psychotic symptoms							
8 Information							
9 Psychological distress							
10 Safety to self							
11 Safety to others							
12 Alcohol							
13 Drugs							
14 Company							
15 Intimate relationships							
16 Sexual expression							
17 Child care							
18 Education							
19 Telephone							
20 Transport							
21 Money							
22 Benefits							

The **met or unmet need** column gives the number of subjects who were rated 1 or 2 in Section 1 of the topic. The **unmet need** column gives the number of subjects who were rated 2 in Section 1 of the topic.

When comparing Section 1 scores (e.g. to analyse reliability) Cohen's κ coefficient (Cohen, 1960) can be used, with standard error in brackets. For some samples, low numbers and a substantial skew in the distribution of ratings will result in misleading κ coefficients (Feinstein & Cicchetti, 1990), in which case percentage agreement will be a better measure to use. When comparing Section 2, 3 and 4 scores, Pearson correlation coefficients can be used, with 95% confidence intervals.

Appendix: Definition of UK-specific examples

Item	Example	Definition
3 Looking after the home	Domestic help	Someone who visits the user's home to perform activities such as cleaning and washing up
4 Self-care	Self-care skills programme	A course organised by staff to help the user to gain skills in self-care
5 Daytime activities	Day centre	A place run by health or social services where users can go during the day and where activities may be organised
8 Information about condition and treatment	MIND	A voluntary organisation promoting the rights of users
11 Safety to others	Anger management programme	Course organised by staff for users with problems in controlling their anger
12 Alcohol	Alcoholics Anonymous	A self-help group for people with alcohol problems
14 Company	Drop-in	Similar to a day centre but less structured
19 Telephone	Phone card	A card containing credit for telephone calls
20 Transport	Bus pass	A card allowing unlimited bus travel for a defined period within a specific area
	Taxi card	Similar to a bus pass

References

Cohen, J. A. (1960) A coefficient of agreement for nominal scales. *Educational and Psychological Measurement*, **20**, 37–46.

Feinstein, A. & Cicchetti, D. (1990) High agreement but low kappa: II. Resolving the paradoxes. *Journal of Clinical Epidemiology*, **43**, 551–558.

Part III

Client Socio-demographic and Service Receipt Inventory – European Version

7 Development of the CSSRI–EU

Daniel Chisholm and Martin Knapp

The clinical and social impacts of schizophrenia on individuals, families and communities include economic consequences (Knapp et al, 1999, 2002). Costs are incurred at all levels of society, either directly through expenditure and unpaid time spent on providing health and social care and support, or indirectly in terms of lost opportunities, such as for leisure or work. The estimation of these costs (derived from description of associated patterns of service uptake or utilisation) is fundamental to comprehensive assessment of the resource consequences of schizophrenia and its treatment; yet standardised methods or instruments for international research have not been developed for this task. Methods for the measurement of service use and costs need to be more sensitive to the local context than do those for rating psychiatric symptoms or assessing behavioural traits and personal abilities. For example, the approach to measurement must take into account the structure or system of treatment and care, and factors relating to patients' access to specific services. The broader socio-economic and cultural contexts will also be relevant, for they will influence, *inter alia*, the prevailing level of unemployment, and the expectations regarding roles of families and wider local communities in supporting people with mental health problems (Johnson et al, 1997).

The aim of the work described in this chapter was to develop an internationally usable method for gathering data on service use and other domains relevant to the economic analysis of mental health care. Specifically, the work represents a core element of the European Psychiatric Services: Inputs Linked to Outcome Domains and Needs (EPSILON) Study, the primary aims of which were to produce standardised versions of instruments in key areas of mental health services research in five European languages, test their reliability, and employ them in a five-country, cross-sectional study of people with schizophrenia (see Chapter 1).

Method

Analytical perspective

For the purposes of mental health economics research, it is desirable to measure service use and costs comprehensively, since the broad personal and social impacts of schizophrenia typically result in a need for contact with many different service agencies, including health services, social services, housing and criminal justice services (Weisbrod et al, 1980; Clark et al, 1994; Knapp et al, 1999). This comprehensive perspective is particularly important for multinational studies, since different countries have established different boundaries between health and other services, and these boundaries have been known to shift over time as a result of changes in government policy or other forces. Also, the balance of responsibilities between the public sector (state) and other agencies may similarly vary from country to country. Data collection should therefore range beyond the immediately observable health service inputs to include other service supports, contacts with other agencies (such as housing and criminal justice) and non-service implications of mental illness (particularly the costs of lost employment and productivity, and the economic burden falling on family caregivers). Moreover, data should be obtained on the frequency and intensity of any service contacts, in order to examine service patterns and to estimate costs accurately.

International research on service utilisation patterns, costs and other economic dimensions of mental health care is complicated by the need to reflect the contexts within which people live and receive their care. Arguably this is true of any research tool, but the problems of economic research that crosses international boundaries are especially acute when the objects of comparison are themselves heavily influenced by social, economic, political, historical and cultural structures and forces peculiar to those countries. To a greater degree than for the other instruments developed in the EPSILON Study, therefore, we needed to ensure that the instruments assessing resource use captured the core features of each of five health care and other systems covered by the study, as well as being sufficiently standardised to permit meaningful international comparison. A core feature was thus to balance local relevance with international generalisability.

Data collection

Selecting the most appropriate method of data capture for economic studies depends on a number of factors, including the primary purpose of the study, the availability of funding and other data collection methods to be used. The main features of the type of study needed to examine service use are in fact quite common in mental health services research:

(a)   a representative sample of people with mental health problems (in this case schizophrenia) treated by 'ordinary' services;

(b)   the aim of making comparisons between samples or sites (in this case, comparisons between countries);

(c)   a cross-sectional design, with the possibility of repeating the observations later on sampled individuals;

(d)   a limited research budget, making it necessary either to rely on extant information sets and/or to collect interview-based data concurrently with clinical and associated data.

The two broad options for data collection that presented themselves were to use existing information held by service-providing or funding agencies, or to rely on individual informants. One of the study sites (Verona) had a psychiatric case register that contained health service utilisation data, and other sites had some electronic data (for example, secondary health care information systems in London and Copenhagen). However, none of the local 'routine information' systems was sufficiently compatible with the others to provide the basis for comparative research. Even if there had been some compatibility, there would be the question of data breadth: do extant systems keep data on all relevant services? We know from previous research that people with schizophrenia use many different services (Knapp *et al*, 1999), so that even if each site had computerised data, they might not cover all relevant services. In the (unlikely) event that they did, there would be the considerable challenge of merging data-sets designed for different health care systems, to meet different local management needs, and using different software. Data capture using electronic information systems was therefore rejected at an early stage. Information on services used by individual people will usually be held by service providers, and some professionals (such as general practitioners) should have a reasonably broad view of service utilisation. The disadvantage of relying on service providers to produce these data is that records or professionals' knowledge will often be incomplete, partial (generally covering only the agency's own responsibilities), and difficult to access or expensive in researcher time. These latter factors were important in this study, and we concluded that we could not rely on agency information holdings in the five sites to provide the range and quality of data needed.

Another way of collecting information is to obtain it directly from individuals, either through interview or a self-completion questionnaire. Postal or self-completion methods (including diary cards) have been used in some previous studies (Mauskopf et al, 1996; Gosden et al, 1997) but were ruled out here, partly because we feared a low response rate, but mainly for the pragmatic reason that other study objectives already required face-to-face interviews, and there is a long tradition of collecting service use and similar information at the same time as clinical data (Beecham, 1995).

Three potential groups of respondents could be interviewed:

(a)   case managers (keyworkers or similar)
(b)   members of the patient's family
(c)   the patients themselves.

A case (or care) manager or keyworker who coordinates services for the patient might be a good respondent, although this would depend on the breadth of the person's responsibilities and knowledge (Widlak et al, 1992). Case management has been implemented in some guise in all of the EPSILON study sites, but because the particular modes of operation and service structures differ in these different sites, standardised reporting of service uptake by case managers would be problematic. When patients live with their family, another data source could be other family members (who may in effect act as informal case managers). In some sites it transpired that a majority of people in the sample lived with at least one relative (72% in Santander, 50% in Verona), but elsewhere this was much less common (20% in Amsterdam and London, and only 4% in Copenhagen). Family members were interviewed for another part of the research study, to complete the Involvement Evaluation Questionnaire (see Chapter 10), but it was felt that this data source was not sufficiently widely available for the purposes of description of service use and cost calculations.

The patient is the only person who is likely to have all or most of the information about which services have been accessed, how often and for how long. However, it is probable that patients will not report service utilisation accurately, either because of their clinical condition, or because they exhibit the common human failing of poor recall. We chose to ask patients for these data, but we needed to take especial care with instrument design to improve the likely accuracy of the information provided (for example, by providing clearly defined and identifiable categories of service or state benefits).

The comparative merits of retrospective and prospective data collection have been discussed elsewhere (Johnston et al, 1998). Prospective data collection essentially requires maintaining a diary of all service contacts, whereas retrospective collection involves occasional completion of an interview, reflecting back on services used in the previous few weeks or months. (Data collection should not be confused with design: prospective trials can of course use retrospective methods for collecting service use data.) In this study, we adopted a 3-month retrospective period, which is sufficiently long to pick up the wide range of services that individuals might take up but without stretching the respondent's powers of recall – there is evidence to suggest that interviewees significantly underreport frequent events when asked to report retrospectively over a 6-month period (Jobe et al, 1990).

Instrument development

The first task was to identify criteria for selection and development of a suitable instrument. Four requirements were identified:

(a)   The instrument should span the domains of accommodation and living circumstances, employment and income, and service utilisation, to allow description of the economic and related circumstances of individual people and the service or care 'packages' that support them.

(b) It should record the frequency and intensity of service use, so that service costs can be calculated as accurately as possible.

(c) After translation, it should be able to be used alongside the other instruments chosen for the EPSILON Study, and it should also be suitable, after only modest adaptation, for use in other European countries.

(d) It should be understandable by respondents (people with schizophrenia) and manageable for use in interviews conducted by trained researchers.

The second stage was to establish whether an existing instrument would meet these requirements. If so, we could move on to its use in the empirical part of the study, examining its performance on samples of people with schizophrenia. If no existing instrument satisfied our requirements, as was the case here, the next task was to develop or adapt one. Rather than start from first principles, we chose to build on an existing instrument, the Client Service Receipt Inventory (CSRI; Beecham & Knapp, 2001). The CSRI has been widely employed and has a multitude of forms, having been used in more than 100 studies since it was first developed in England in the mid-1980s). Although it has been used outside the UK, the CSRI has not previously been subjected to the degree of developmental work or scrutiny employed in this study. In particular, close attention was paid to the categorisation of housing, employment and service use items of the inventory in order to generate an instrument capable of international use (see below).

A set of baseline questions was generated which covered the topics of interest (initially in English, subsequently translated into the other four languages). This baseline schedule was then subjected to a process of cross-cultural validation and refinement, based on the discussions in focus groups at each site (see Chapter 2). The final stage in the development of this instrument was to administer it to a sample of individuals at each site, and further revise it in the light of any difficulties or misinterpretation.

The form of the instrument

The Client Socio-demographic and Service Receipt Inventory – European Version (CSSRI–EU) is constructed around five main sections: socio-demographic information, usual living situation, employment and income, service receipt and medication profile.

Socio-demographic information

A range of categorised socio-demographic variables, including date of birth, gender, marital status, ethnic group, mother tongue, years of schooling and level of educational attainment comprise the initial section of the instrument. Although some of these variables (such as age or gender) appear in other instruments, these data were comprehensively recorded here for completeness. Moreover, such data lead naturally on to consideration of other socio-economic circumstances.

Usual living situation

Accommodation represents an important parameter for economic studies of mental disorder, largely because of the high cost of specialist residential care. An individual's living situation (alone, in a family or living with other, non-related residents) is also a potentially significant predictor of cost (and outcomes). Accommodation was divided into domestic, hospital and community residential categories, each with clearly defined sub-categories (for example, tenure of domestic accommodation or staffing cover/ intensity in residential care). Changes in accommodation over the retrospective period can be recorded.

For people resident in non-domestic accommodation, completion of a one-page supplement was requested, containing information on the number of (available and occupied) places/beds in the facility, the total complement and cost of care staff, other revenue costs and the average weekly charge or fee per resident place/bed. This supplement, based on a schedule developed for costing mental health residential care in the UK (Chisholm et al, 1997), was an addition to the original CSRI and was completed after the face-to-face interview, in consultation with a facility manager. It was not part of the interview with the patient, and would not be needed if unit cost data were to be drawn from an established source rather than calculated anew.

Employment and income

Information about patients' employment and income is important for establishing the indirect costs and effects of schizophrenia, such as lost days of work, and also for estimating the living expenses of the patient. Employment status was divided into a number of appropriate categories (paid or self-employed, unemployed, housewife/husband, etc.); occupational categories were based on an international standard classification of occupations (manager/administrator, professional, skilled labourer, etc.). The approach taken regarding state benefits was to identify a number of international categories of benefits or entitlements (unemployment and income support; sickness and disability; housing; other), and to have a list of national variants that fell under these broad categories (for example, 'jobseekers' allowance' in the UK). This enabled us both to make consistent comparisons between study sites and to build up a set of data that has most meaning and use within each individual site. Personal (gross) income was also requested, using bands obtained from national statistics bureaux that reflect the quintiles of gross income in each country (so that the proportions of patients falling into these internationally equivalent income bands could be compared).

Service receipt

A range of psychiatric, social and general medical services were identified which together were considered to make up a comprehensive profile of services available to the patient population in each of the five centres. The main categories were: psychiatric and general medical in-patient hospital admissions and total days; psychiatric and general medical hospital out-patient attendances; community-based day services (frequency and intensity of attendance); and contacts with primary care, social services and community mental health care professionals. Clear definitions were attached to individual service components or categories, in order to be able to compare the different sites, and space was left for inclusion of other services provided to patients that were not specifically identified in the inventory. For each service, the numbers of contacts in the previous 3 months were requested, and, where applicable, the sector of provision (statutory/government, voluntary or private). A final subsection asked for contact with criminal justice services (number of police contacts, nights in custody, psychiatric assessments or court appearances).

Medication profile

A profile of the individual's use of all prescribed medications in the previous month was requested, incorporating the name of the drug, the dosage level and frequency, and whether it was prescribed on a depot basis.

Translations and focus groups

Once the baseline version of the instrument had been developed, the next steps were translation into the other four European languages (Danish, Dutch, Italian, Spanish), by either professional translators or local researchers, followed by cross-cultural validation of the translated instrument. Since the CSSRI–EU is an inventory of socio-economic indicators and service variables rather than a multi-item rating scale of a particular outcome domain, the focus in this study was on achieving face validity and semantic equivalence within and between individual participating sites, rather than formal exploration of the reliability of the measure between raters, sites or time points (see Chapter 3). This took place through both informal dialogue and discussion with principal investigators and other interested parties, and more formally through the conduct of focus groups. Focus groups consisted of between six and ten individuals (psychiatrists, other health professionals, social care workers, informal carers and service users), and were intended to address two aspects of the instrument: its content and its language (see Chapter 2).

The CSSRI–EU focus groups generated a number of system-level comments that revolved around the perceived incompatibility of national health, social and welfare structures with the attempted European-wide structures or categories given in the initial version of the CSSRI–EU. These comments related to two sections of the instrument: usual living situation, and employment and income. In particular, focus groups suggested reordering the categories of employment, benefit entitlements and accommodation so as to reflect their own national systems better. These suggestions were incorporated as far as possible, without losing the core requirement of inter-site comparability. For example, four international categories of state benefits were developed (unemployment/income support; sickness/ disability; housing; pension), within which sites could specify local variants of these broader categories. Residential care was a further area that required reordering, owing to the heterogeneity of service arrangements in different sites. This problem was overcome by describing the final categories in neutral, broad terms (overnight facility, 24-hour staffed; overnight facility, staffed (not 24 hours); overnight facility, unstaffed).

A second set of comments revolved around country-specific suggestions for enhancing the understanding, definition or measurement of individual items or components included in the service receipt section of the inventory. A particular area of discussion concerned the appropriate classification and definition of day care and support facilities and community-based mental health services. For example, the Dutch system of community mental health centres needed to be correctly classified under the appropriate item in the inventory.

The instrument was then revised, both in its original English form (in the light of focus group recommendations as to content) and in each of four translations (in the light of recommendations about terminology or language).

Exploratory use of the instrument

The CSSRI–EU was now ready for use in empirical research. In this study the sample was selected in each of the five sites by employing the same diagnostic and administrative criteria (adults aged 18–65 years inclusive with an ICD–10 diagnosis of schizophrenia: code F20). All patients had been in contact with mental health services during the 3-month period preceding the start of the study (see Chapter 1). Fieldwork was conducted over 15 months in the five sites. For each service itemised in the CSSRI–EU, unit costs were calculated in each site to cover salaries of staff employed in direct patient care and management, facility operating costs, plus overhead and capital costs. Unit costs were converted into UK pounds using 'purchasing power parities', which are rates of currency conversion that eliminate price-level differences between countries (these are routinely calculated by the Organization for

Economic Cooperation and Development, in collaboration with the Statistical Office of the European Community). The main findings regarding service use and costs for this sample are reported elsewhere (Chisholm & Knapp, 2002; Knapp *et al*, 2002), but a number of methodological issues that emerged in the course of data collection and in the following initial examination of the final data-set can be summarised here.

First, the response rate in terms of completion of the CSSRI–EU was 100%; no refusal to be interviewed was encountered across the sites. This unusually high response rate may be attributable in part to the integration of service utilisation questions with key socio-demographic characteristics (the latter being of fundamental importance to analyses, over and above economic evaluation). Response rates to individual items within the CSSRI–EU were also high (where applicable), indicating few difficulties of interpretation. For items or services not available in, or not applicable to, a site (for example, long-stay psychiatric wards in certain sites), zero was entered for all cases.

Structured response categories for a range of socio-demographic and socio-economic indicators (such as living situation, level of educational attainment and state benefit entitlements) performed well. The only clear source of inter-site differences in interpretation related to employment status: specifically, the classification of patients not in open or sheltered employment; in certain sites, such patients were categorised as 'unemployed', whereas in other sites a large proportion were classified as 'retired', in the sense that they were in receipt of a disability allowance or pension and were not expected or likely to be employed in the future.

As expected, and allowed for in the baseline version of the instrument, a number of specific services had been used over and above those specified. These service contacts were recorded as an 'other service' under the appropriate service category, together with a brief text description of the service, and subsequently recoded or described in their own right. For one site (Verona), where the same professionals provide both hospital and community care (continuity of care model), there was evidence of 'double counting' of service provision, which subsequently required checking of CSSRI–EU data with that centre's psychiatric case register. A final area of difficulty experienced in the service receipt section of the instrument was coding of the dosage frequency for prescribed medications, because sites adopted different approaches for recording frequency rates for depot v. other drugs.

On the basis of these analyses, a final set of revisions was made to the instrument (and accompanying manual) in order for it to be usable in other research studies. For example, specific services included under 'other' for a particular service category were incorporated as necessary, and guidance was modified for coding employment status and frequency of medication use.

Discussion

From the outset of the EPSILON Study it was agreed that one part of the empirical study should look at economic aspects of schizophrenia care. After considering a number of methodological options, we developed an instrument – the CSSRI–EU – for use in interviews with patients and/or key staff. The CSSRI–EU is easy to use after a short amount of interviewer training (1–2 hours; the brief manual also provides guidance on completion), can be completed in interviews by people with schizophrenia, takes only about 20 minutes to complete, and provides information useful for a number of evaluative and other purposes both within and across countries. The CSSRI–EU enables us to trace patterns of service use and care in an international context, calculate the associated costs of care, and examine relationships or differences across countries between costs and a range of socio-demographic and clinical characteristics. Each of these capabilities can be usefully employed to improve the planning, provision and evaluation of mental health services for people with schizophrenia.

Since the CSSRI–EU is an inventory of variables required for economic analysis, rather than a multi-item rating scale, the focus of the development process was on achieving face validity within and between individual participating sites, rather than formal exploration of the reliability of the measure between raters, sites or time points. The absence of such reliability measures represents a gap in our understanding of how accurate the CSSRI–EU is in recording rates of service use. Although significant but relatively uncommon events such as hospitalisation are readily remembered, there is concern that reports by patients of the frequency and intensity of their contact with community-based service professionals is subject to recall error (Jobe *et al*, 1990; Clark *et al*, 1994; Johnston *et al*, 1998). This possible source of error can be examined by comparing the values given by patients in the CSSRI–EU with an alternative data source, either another informant (an informal carer or keyworker) or an administrative database. We have already commented on the limitations of these alternative sources of data in an international context, specifically the incomplete knowledge of other informants and the absence of standardised, high-quality information systems across countries. Where they exist, however, well-maintained psychiatric case registers do represent one important data source against which to assess the performance of certain elements of service receipt schedules such as the CSSRI–EU. Such an analysis was not an objective of this study, but recent work in one of the sites (Verona) has considered these issues and showed that the agreement on overall psychiatric costs was high: the concordance correlation coefficient was 0.93 for all patients and 0.97 for patients with a diagnosis of schizophrenia (Mirandola *et al*, 1999).

References

Beecham, J. K. (1995) Collecting and estimating costs. In *The Economic Evaluation of Mental Health Services* (ed. M. R. J. Knapp). Aldershot: Ashgate.

Beecham, J. K. & Knapp, M. R. J. (2001) Costing psychiatric interventions. In *Measuring Mental Health Needs* (2nd edn) (eds G. Thornicroft, C. Brewin & J. K. Wing). London: Gaskell.

Chisholm, D. & Knapp, M. R. J. (2002) The economics of schizophrenia care in Europe: the EPSILON study. *Epidemiologia e Psichiatria*, **11**, 12–17.

Chisholm, D., Knapp, M. R. J., Astin, J., et al (1997) The mental health residential care study: the costs of provision. *Journal of Mental Health*, **6**, 85–99.

Clark, R. E., Teague, G. B., Ricketts, S. K., et al (1994) Measuring resource use in economic evaluations: determining the social costs of mental illness. *Journal of Mental Health Administration*, **21**, 32–41.

Gosden, T. B., Black, M. E., Mead, N. J., et al (1997) The efficiency of specialist outreach clinics in general practice: is further evaluation needed? *Journal of Health Services Research and Policy*, **3**, 177–179.

Jobe, J. B., White, A. A., Kelley, C. L., et al (1990) Recall strategies and memory of health care visits. *Millbank Quarterly*, **68**, 171–189.

Johnson, S., Ramsay, R. & Thornicroft, G. (1997) Londoners' mental health needs: the sociodemographic context. In *London's Mental Health: The Report to the King's Fund London Commission* (eds S. Johnson, R. Ramsay & G. Thornicroft). London: King's Fund.

Johnston, K., Buxton, M., Jones, D. R., et al (1998) *Assessing the Costs of Health Care Technologies in Clinical Trials. Final report to the Health Technology Assessment Programme.* Uxbridge: Brunel University, Health Economics Research Group.

Knapp, M. R. J., Almond, S. & Percudani, M. (1999) Costs of schizophrenia. In *Evidence and Experience in Psychiatry* (eds M. Maj & N. Sartorius). Geneva: World Psychiatric Association.

Knapp, M. R. J., Chisholm, D., Leese, M., et al (2002) Comparing patterns and costs of schizophrenia care in five European countries: the EPSILON Study. *Acta Psychiatrica Scandinavica*, **105**, 42–54.

Mauskopf, J., Schulman, K., Bell, L., et al (1996) A strategy for collecting pharmacoeconomic data during phase II/III clinical trials. *Pharmacoeconomics*, **9**, 264–277.

Mirandola, M., Bisoffi, G., Bonizzato, P., et al (1999) Collecting psychiatric resources utilisation data to calculate costs of care. A comparison between a service receipt interview and a case register. *Social Psychiatry and Psychiatric Epidemiology*, **34**, 541–547.

Weisbrod, B. A., Test, M. A. & Stein, L. I. (1980) Alternatives to mental hospital treatment: II. Economic benefit– cost analysis. *Archives of General Psychiatry*, **37**, 400–405.

Widlak, P. A., Greenley, J. R. & McKee, D. (1992) Validity of case manager reports of clients' functioning in the community: independent living, income, employment, family contact and problem behaviours. *Community Mental Health Journal*, **28**, 505–517.

8 Introduction and manual for the CSSRI–EU

Daniel Chisholm and Martin Knapp

The Client Socio-demographic and Service Receipt Inventory – European version (CSSRI–EU) is one of five instruments developed to measure the needs, quality of life and costs of schizophrenia in five European countries: Denmark, England, Italy, the Netherlands and Spain. The CSSRI–EU brings together questions that allow the comprehensive costing of care packages for individuals with schizophrenia; it does this by collecting information on the current living arrangements and expenses of the individual (including income, employment and accommodation), followed by questions about any use the person might have made of a range of health care, social care and other services over a defined retrospective period. A profile of the person's medication is compiled in a similar way. Unit costs for each of these services and drugs (calculated as a separate procedure) are then applied to derive the total cost associated with the individual's use of services and medication. The CSSRI–EU is also used to collect socio-demographic data. Costs associated with the informal care inputs by family and friends are assessed using a different instrument, the Involvement Evaluation Questionnaire (see Chapter 10).

This chapter provides explanatory notes for items in the CSSRI–EU that might require additional information, definition or guidance.

Contact point

Further information can be obtained from Professor Martin Knapp at the Centre for the Economics of Mental Health, PO29, Health Services Research Department, David Goldberg Centre, Institute of Psychiatry, De Crespigny Park, London SE5 8AF, UK. Tel: +44 (0)20 7848 0198; e-mail: cemh@iop.kcl.ac.uk.

Explanatory notes

Front page: patient's confidential details

This page is to be completed at the beginning of the face-to-face interview. It should be stored securely in a separate location to the completed schedule, in order to preserve the confidentiality of the interview.

Patient number

Please ensure that this is recorded before the interview begins.

Date of birth

Complete here on the front page and also on the main instrument (Q 1.1) so that the person can be traced even if the patient number is illegible.

Section 1: socio-demographic information

Q 1.4 Ethnic group

It was not possible to generate a coded shortlist of possible ethnic groups, as the CSSRI–EU was designed to be used in five different countries, each with its own historical, political and cultural heritage.

'Ethnicity' is defined as 'shared origins, social background, traditions or culture that lead to a sense of identity and group'. The ethnic group of most patients in the EPSILON Study was best described as 'White European': other possibilities included 'African–Caribbean', 'Sikh' and 'Chinese'. Ethnicity is not to be confused with 'race', which is the categorisation of people by their physical characteristics.

Q 1.5 Country of birth

Country of birth is an objective (but potentially crude) index of ethnicity.

Q 1.7 Years of schooling

The starting point is the beginning of compulsory (free) schooling.

Section 2: Living situation

Q 2.1 Usual living situation

Please identify in consultation with the respondent his or her usual place of residence. (Definition of children: young people under 18 years old.)

Q 2.2 Type of accommodation

This item attempts to provide a simple classification of possible types of accommodation. Some of the categories are necessarily broad in order to allow comparisons to be made between different countries. The following definitions should be used to categorise specialist community and hospital accommodation:

- Overnight facility, 24-hour staffed: facility where a member of staff is present on site 24 hours a day, with responsibilities related to the monitoring and clinical and social care of patients (i.e. not domestic or security staff).
- Overnight facility, staffed (not 24-hour): a member of staff is regularly on site at least 3 days a week for some part of the day, with responsibilities related to the monitoring and clinical and social care of patients.
- Overnight facility, unstaffed: staff are on site fewer than 3 days a week, i.e. staff are present only occasionally during the week, either on a regular visit or in response to particular care needs.

- Acute psychiatric ward: acute facility to which patients are routinely admitted because of a deterioration in mental state, behaviour or social functioning that is related to a psychiatric disorder.
- Rehabilitation ward: non-acute facility to which patients are referred, usually for a fixed maximum period of residence.
- Long-stay ward: non-acute facility to which patients are referred, usually for an indefinite period.
- General medical ward: facility having the core function of caring for in-patients who do not have a psychiatric disorder.

If the respondent is living in hospital or specialist community accommodation, it is necessary to complete the supplementary page of the schedule (after the interview with the patient), which asks for facility staffing and financial details (see below).

Section 3: Employment and income

Information about the respondent's employment and income is important in establishing the 'knock-on' effects (or indirect costs) of schizophrenia, such as lost ability to work, and also for estimating the living expenses of the respondent.

Q 3.2 Occupational categories

The categories are based on the International Standard Classification of Occupations (ISCO).

Q 3.4 State benefits

The approach taken here has been to identify a number of international categories of benefits and entitlements, and to list the national variants that fall into these categories. This meets the dual requirement of enabling consistent comparisons between countries, while building up a set of data that have most meaning and use in each individual country.

Q 3.6 Personal income

We have attempted to reduce the sensitivity of questions about personal income by offering a number of possible income bands. These can be listed on a separate card which is shown to the respondent, who is asked to point to the number of the band that corresponds to their total personal income (per week, per month or per year – it does not matter which, each amounts to the same income level). If possible this should be given as gross income (i.e. before tax and other deductions); otherwise the net income level can be recorded (i.e. after tax and deductions). Please note that this question asks for the income of the individual respondent, not household income. Currency should be expressed in local units and can be converted from UK pounds sterling (in the UK version reproduced in this book) by applying official exchange rates.

Section 4: Service receipt

Service receipts are collected for a retrospective period of 3 months, with the exception of hospital in-patient services which are recorded for a period of 12 months.

Q 4.1 In-patient hospital services

Please record all days spent in these facilities, over a period of 12 months. These should be recorded even if the respondent was identified as currently living in such a facility (Q 2.2). The categories of facility are defined above.

Q 4.3 Community-based day services

This item applies to services that are normally available to several patients at a time and that usually provide some combination of treatment for problems related to mental illness, structured activity, and social contact or support. These facilities have regular opening hours.

Q 4.4 Primary and community care contacts

Primary and community care services involve contact between health and social care professionals and patients for some purpose related to management of mental illness and its associated clinical and social difficulties. They are provided separately, i.e. they do not form part of the delivery of residential or day services.

    Please identify the sector from which the service contact is delivered: 1, statutory or government; 2, voluntary; 3, private. If there is a mixture of sectors for any given contact, indicate the main sector of provision.

Q 4.5 Criminal justice services

Code as '9' if the number of police contacts, nights in custody, psychiatric assessments or court appearances is not known.

Section 5: Medication profile

Q 5.1 Medication

Record all drugs taken, not just those related to mental illness. Code as '9' if dosage not known, otherwise give amounts in milligrams (e.g. 5 mg).

Supplement: Hospital or community accommodation details

The final page of the schedule needs to be completed only for respondents who are living in hospital or specialist community settings, rather than domestic accommodation. Data should be collected after the face-to-face interview, in consultation with a facility manager or senior keyworker. We recommend that time is made available for this as soon after the patient interview as possible.

    If several respondents are living in the same facility the accommodation details will need to obtained only once; however, please ensure that these details are recorded on each respondent's schedule.

Q 1 Number of places/beds

Record the number of places in the residential facility or hospital ward that are both currently available and occupied.

Q 2 Staffing

Include all staff involved in the direct care and management of patients. The number of full-time equivalent (FTE) staff is calculated by aggregating all full-time and part-time positions and expressing them in terms of full-time posts. For example, a facility with four full-time posts and four half-time posts would have an FTE count of six. The total annual costs of the various categories of staff should include actual salaries only – salary on-costs, such as national insurance, will be calculated separately by CEMH.

Q 3 Recurrent costs (excluding care staff)

Apart from the salaries of care workers, there are other revenue or recurrent costs involved with operating the facility. Using annual accounts (if available), identify the annual costs associated with catering and cleaning staff and consumables, heating and lighting, transport, etc. For hospital wards, an apportionment of the overall hospital recurrent costs (excluding care staff) may be the best estimate possible.

Do not include costs such as rent, capital allowances or overheads; these are a relatively small proportion of the overall cost and should be calculated separately by CEMH.

(If you do have useful information about these costs that you can share with us, please contact Martin Knapp at CEMH.)

Q 4 Charge per week

The charge per week is the fee or price that is payable in the market for residential care. It is often different from the actual cost of the resources involved in residential or hospital care, such as staffing or running costs. For example, a private, for-profit company might charge a fee above what it actually costs to provide care. Fees or charges for a place at a facility are often available, and are useful when it is difficult to estimate the true cost.

9 Client Socio-demographic and Service Receipt Inventory – European Version

Daniel Chisholm and Martin Knapp

Client Socio-demographic and Service Receipt Inventory – European Version (CSSRI–EU)

Centre/Country _____ Patient study number ☐☐☐ Date (dd/mm/yy) ☐☐/☐☐/☐☐

1 Socio-demographic information

1.1 Date of birth (dd/mm/yy/) Date: ☐☐/☐☐/☐☐

1.2 Gender
1 Female
2 Male ☐

1.3 Marital status
1 Single/unmarried
2 Married
3 Separated
4 Divorced
5 Widow/widower
9 Not known ☐

1.4 What is your ethnic group? _____

1.5 Country of birth Country: _____

1.6 Mother tongue
1 National language
2 Other language (but **good** knowledge of national language)
3 Other language (and **poor** or **no** knowledge of national language) ☐

1.7 Number of years in schooling in **general** education Years: ☐☐

1.8 Highest completed level of education
1 Primary level or less
2 Secondary level
3 Tertiary/further education
4 Other general education
9 Not known ☐

1.9 What **further** education or vocational training have you completed or are doing now? *(Tick all boxes that apply)*
☐ Specific vocational training (<1 year)
☐ Specific vocational training (>1 year)
☐ Tertiary level qualification/diploma
☐ University degree (undergraduate)
☐ University higher degree (postgraduate)
☐ Other vocational training

2   Usual living situation

2.1   What is your usual/normal living situation now?

1 Living alone (+/– children)
2 Living with husband/wife (+/–children)
3 Living together as a couple
4 Living with parents
5 Living with other relatives
6 Living with others
9 Not known

2.2   What kind of accommodation is it?
(Refer to manual for directions)

Domestic/family

1 Owner-occupied flat or house
2 Privately rented flat or house
3 Rented from local authority/municipality or housing association/cooperative

Community (non-hospital)

4 Overnight facility, 24-hour staffed
5 Overnight facility, staffed (not 24-hour)
6 Overnight facility, unstaffed at all times

Hospital

7 Acute psychiatric ward
8 Rehabilitation psychiatric ward
9 Long-stay psychiatric ward
10 General medical ward

11 Homeless/roofless

12 Other _____

2.3   If **domestic** accommodation

How many adults live there?
(over the age of 18)

Number of adults

And how many children?
(under the age of 18)

Number of children

Note: if hospital or community accommodation:
Complete the final sheet of the schedule after finishing this interview.

2.4   Have you lived anywhere else in the past 12 months?

1 Yes
2 No

If yes: please complete table:

Accommodation type (See Q 2.2 for code)	Number of days in past 12 months

3   Employment and income

3.1   What is your employment status?

1 Paid or self-employed
2 Voluntary employment
3 Sheltered employment
4 Unemployed
5 Student
6 Housewife/husband
7 Retired
8 Other _____

3.2   **If employed**: state occupation

1 Manager/administrator
2 Professional *(e.g. health, teaching, legal)*
3 Associate professional *(e.g. technical, nursing)*
4 Clerical worker/secretary
5 Skilled labourer *(e.g. building, electrical)*
6 Services/sales *(e.g. retail)*
7 Factory worker
8 Other _____

How many days have you been absent from work owing to illness within the past 3 months?

Number of days:

3.3   **If unemployed:**

Number of weeks unemployed within the past 3 months

Number of weeks:

3.4   Do you receive any state benefits?

1 Yes
2 No

If yes, what benefits are received?
(Please tick all boxes that apply)

International categories	**National variants**
Unemployment/income support	Income support
	Jobseeker's allowance
Sickness/disability	Disability living allowance
	Statutory sick pay
Housing	Housing benefit
Other benefits	State pension
	Child benefit

3.5   What is your **main** income source?

1 Salary/wage
2 State benefits
3 Pension
4 Family support *(e.g. from spouse)*

3.6   What is your total personal **gross** income from all sources?

(Note: if gross income is not known, please give net income, i.e. after tax and other deductions)

	Weekly *or*	**Monthly** *or*	**Yearly**
1	Under £149	Less than £649	Less than £7785
2	£150–£204	£650–£885	£7786–£10 635
3	£205–£279	£886–£1208	£10 636–£14 504
4	£280–£392	£1209–£1699	£14 505–£20 394
5	More than £393	More than £1700	More than £20 395

Gross income ☐   or Net income ☐

4   Service receipt

4.1   Please list any use of **in-patient hospital services** over the past 12 months

(Note1: please enter '0' if service has not been used. Note 2: see manual for definitions)

Service	Admissions	Total number of in-patient days (over past 12 months)
Acute psychiatric ward		
Psychiatric rehabilitation ward		
Long-stay ward		
Emergency/crisis centre		
General medical ward		
Other _____		

4.2   Please list any use of **out-patient hospital services** over the past 3 months

(Note 1: please enter '0' if service has not been used. Note 2: see manual for definitions)

Service	Unit of measurement	Number of units received (over the past 3 months)
Psychiatric out-patient visit	Appointment	
Other hospital out-patient visit (including A&E)	Appointment	
Day hospital	Day attendance	
Other _____		

4.3   Please list any use of **community-based day services** over the past 3 months

(Note 1: please enter '0' if service has not been used. Note 2: see manual for definitions)

Service	Number of attendances	Average duration of attendance
Community mental health centre		
Day care centre		
Group therapy		
Sheltered workshop		
Specialist education		
Other _____		

4.4   Please list any other **primary and secondary community care contacts** over the past 3 months
       (Note 1: please enter '0' if service has not been used. Note 2: see manual for definitions)

Service	Sector (1=govt; 2=vol.; 3=private)	Total number of contacts over the past 3 months	Average contact time (minutes)
Psychiatrist			
Psychologist			
Primary care physician			
District nurse			
Community psychiatric nurse/ case manager			
Social worker			
Occupational therapist			
Home help/care worker			
Other _____			
Other _____			

4 .5   Over the past 3 months, has the patient   1 Yes
       been in contact with the **criminal justice**   2 No
       services?

       If yes, how many contacts with the police?   Number of contacts
       (Note: contact=interview or stay of some hours,
       but not overnight)

       How many nights spent in a police cell or prison?   Number of nights

       How many psychiatric assessments while   Number of assessments
       in custody?

       How many (criminal or civil) court appearances?   Criminal courts

                                                        Civil courts

5   Medication profile

5.1   Please list below use of **any** drugs taken over the past **one month**

Name of drug	Dosage (if known)	Dosage frequency	Depot (1=yes; 0=no)
1.			
2.			
3.			
4.			
5.			

Client Socio-demographic and Service Receipt Inventory – European Version (CSSRI–EU)

Centre/ Country _____   Patient study number ☐☐☐   Date (dd/mm/yy) ☐☐/☐☐/☐☐

Hospital or community accommodation details

*Note: this sheet should be completed as soon as possible **after** the patient face-to-face interview. The best source of information is likely to be a keyworker or facility manager.*

1. How many beds/places in the hospital ward or residential facility are currently available and occupied?

    Available beds/places ☐☐☐

    Occupied beds/places ☐☐☐

2. Please complete the following staffing tables *(see manual for assistance):*

Care staff category *(Note: only one category per staff member)*	Number of full-time equivalent posts	Total annual cost of care staff category
Staff with a medical qualification		
Staff with a psychology qualification		
Staff with a nursing qualification		
Staff with a social care qualification		
Staff with no care qualification		
Vacant care staff positions		
All care staff categories (total)		

3. What is the annual recurrent cost of the facility, excluding care staff? *(Include catering, cleaning, etc., but exclude rent and capital costs; see manual)*

    Total cost per year   £ _____

4. What is the average weekly charge or fee per resident place/bed? *(See manual for definition)*

    Charge per week   £ _____

5. Who contributes towards the full cost of this accommodation? *(Tick all boxes that apply)*

    National government (health service/insurance fund)   ☐

    Local government   ☐

    Voluntary organisation/charity   ☐

    Private organisation/company   ☐

    Private individual   ☐

Part IV

Involvement Evaluation Questionnaire – European Version

10 Introduction and manual for the IEQ–EU

Aart Schene, Bob van Wijngaarden and Maarten Koeter

The Involvement Evaluation Questionnaire – European Version (IEQ–EU) was developed to measure the consequences of mental illness for family members and others caring for someone with schizophrenia. This chapter describes the questionnaire, how and when it should be used, and its applicability.

Some terminology

The consequences of mental illness for family members have been described in a variety of ways. Treudley (1946) was the first to use the term 'burden on the family', referring to the consequences for those in close contact with a severely disturbed patient with a psychiatric disorder. Later terms used were 'burden on the community' (Sainsbury & Grad, 1962), 'disturbance caused by the patient' (Brown & Rutter, 1966) and 'the presence of problems, difficulties or adverse events, which affect the lives of psychiatric patients' significant others, e.g. members of the household or the family' (Platt, 1985). More recently 'caregiving' has been considered to be a more appropriate term, because it lacks the negative and stigmatising connotation of 'burden' or 'disturbance', and covers all possible positive and negative consequences of mental disorders for family members (Szmukler, 1996; Joyce *et al*, 2000). In this chapter we also use the term 'caregiving consequences'.

Families and mental illness: the domains

The influence of mental illness on family members can be understood and summarised as a series of interconnected domains (Creer *et al*, 1982; Fadden, 1984; Schene, 1986, 1990; van Wijngaarden *et al*, 2003).

Symptoms and symptomatic behaviour

The severity of symptoms and symptomatic behaviour were found to be an important factor in caregiver consequences. This was particularly evident for aggressive and hostile behaviour, self-destructive behaviour (suicide attempts and self-mutilation), negative symptoms, sleep disturbance, addiction to medication, alcohol or illegal drugs, mood swings and dysphoria, hallucinations, delusions and paranoia.

In addition, difficulties in terms of role dysfunction such as lack of social contacts, poor hygiene and lack of household responsibilities are important.

Caring and coping

When people with mental illness are unable to do what could normally be expected of them, others have to take over these tasks, which can be burdensome. These caregiver consequences were described by Gubman *et al* (1987) as *do's* and *don'ts*: the *do's* were the extra tasks caregivers had to do, and the *don'ts* were activities they were no longer able to do because of the caregiving tasks.

Family relations

The psychiatric symptoms and disruptive behaviour of the affected person and the resulting caring tasks may cause relationships between other family members to become strained. Some caregivers described their experience as a sense of loss of the premorbid personality, with all its characteristics and promises, and the loss of hopes, dreams and expectations (Miller *et al*, 1990).

Household routine and family functioning

The caregiving tasks in combination with the patient's symptomatic behaviour sometimes lead to quarrels and distress which may have a great impact on family and marital relationships. Family systems may break up and marital relationships may end in divorce.

Social relations and stigmatisation

The social networks of families caring for a relative with a chronic disorder often decline. This may result in family members becoming more vulnerable to psychiatric problems themselves. It is not only patients who are stigmatised; the caregivers suffer too.

Leisure time and career

Like social relationships, opportunities for pursuing hobbies, sports, club activities, recreation and holidays also decline. Some caregivers have to stop working, or have to accept reduced career prospects.

Finances

The financial position of the family may deteriorate because caregivers have to quit work. This may be exacerbated by the extra expenses incurred, for example for medical or psychiatric care, or by the need to support the patient financially.

Children and siblings

Growing up with a parent or sibling with a mental illness may put at risk the healthy psychological development of the child (Beisser *et al*, 1967; Beardslee *et al*, 1983).

Mental health care system

Many caregivers have reported burdensome contacts with the mental health care system. There was a lack of information about the origin of the disorder and its prognosis, on how to cope, on medication and its side-effects, and on the availability of services in times of crisis.

Subjective distress

Caring for a relative with mental illness may lead to feelings of guilt, uncertainty, ambivalence, hate, anger, sympathy, withdrawal, depression, anxiety, hopelessness, chronic sorrow and bereavement.

Caregiver's health

The subjective distress described above, together with the disruption to family life and the stress of caregiving tasks, may have consequences for both the physical and mental health of the caregiver. New mental health problems may emerge, and existing problems may be exacerbated.

Positive experiences

In recent years attention has also been paid to possible positive consequences of caregiving. Caring for a relative or friend with mental illness could lead to positive personal experiences and good aspects of the relationship, such as discovering one's own strength, feeling closer to the patient or others, feeling useful, and enjoying the patient's presence (Szmukler *et al*, 1996; Joyce *et al*, 2000).

Objective and subjective consequences

A distinction between the objective and subjective aspects of caregiving is made in the literature (Platt, 1985). Objective aspects are directly connected to the patient's symptoms, symptomatic behaviour and social functioning; they include things that caregivers have to do (helping, supervising, controlling, paying, etc.) or are now unable to do (hobbies clubs, career, work) as a consequence of the caregiving task; objective consequences are the 'time and effort required for one person to attend to the needs of another' (Biegel *et al*, 1991). Subjective consequences relate to caregivers' short-term and long-term reactions to the symptoms and behavioural characteristics of the patient and the caregiving tasks arising from them. Perceived distress and interpersonal strain are examples of short-term reactions; they refer to the stress of everyday caregiving. These short-term reactions may lead to more enduring consequences, with an impact on overall well-being, satisfaction with life, physical and mental health, social isolation, divorce and family disintegration.

Several models have been formulated to clarify the relationship between objective and subjective caregiving consequences, and the effect of mediating variables (Maurin & Barmann, 1990; Schene, 1990; Biegel *et al*, 1991; Gallop *et al*, 1991). These models are mostly stress–coping–support–appraisal models. Objective consequences are considered as independent variables and subjective consequences as dependent variables, mediated by individual, familial, societal and cultural variables (Schene, 1990). Examples of mediating variables are caregiver's coping style and relationship with the patient, social support, the quality and quantity of the local mental health care system, and culturally dependent ideologies and philosophies about mental illness and caregiving. The models that have been formulated indicate that there will not be a simple, straightforward relationship between patient characteristics, the objective consequences of caregiving and the resulting subjective consequences. For example, caregivers who are able to cope with their caring role, who receive help from friends and relatives and who feel supported by mental health professionals will probably be less prone to long-term subjective consequences than caregivers who are unable to cope and who feel isolated, stigmatised and misunderstood.

Structure and content of the IEQ–EU

The questionnaire consists of seven modules, each of which can be used separately.

Demographic factors

Socio-demographic characteristics and contact details for the respondent and the respondent's family are elicited by items 1–15; these include age, gender, household composition and number of hours of contact between patient and caregiver.

Caregiving consequences

Caregiving consequences of psychiatric disorders (items 16–46) form the core module of the IEQ–EU, with items referring to all kinds of encouragement and care that the caregiver has to give to the patient, supervision of the patient's dangerous behaviours, interpersonal problems between patient and caregiver, caregiver's worrying, and caregiver's coping and subjective burden. All items are scored in a five-point Likert scale (0 'never', 1 'sometimes', 2 'regularly', 3 'often', 4 'always'). Most items relate to the 4 weeks prior to assessment ('How often during the past 4 weeks have you helped –'), but items 44–46 have no specified time frame.

Expenses

Items 47–54 identify additional financial costs incurred on behalf of the patient, for instance for professional help, to pay for damage caused by the patient's behaviour, or for financial support in case of unemployment.

Psychological distress

Between 1992 and 1997 this module consisted of an eight-item scale referring to psychosomatic or somatic complaints such as sleeplessness, irritability and feelings of depression. In 1997 this scale was replaced by the 12-item General Health Questionnaire (GHQ–12; Goldberg & Williams, 1988) as a measure of caregiver distress.

Need for professional help

Items 67–69 deal with the caregiver's use of professional help for psychosomatic or somatic complaints.

Children

Consequences for the patient's children (under 16 years old) are investigated in items 70–80; these cover difficulties such as loss of appetite, sleeplessness and behavioural problems.

Open question

Item 81 is an open question for the caregiver's own remarks and additions.

Sub-scales

Twenty-seven items in the core module can be summarised into four sub-scales: 'tension' (items 29–35, 42, 43); 'urging' (items 16–21,27, 28); 'worrying' (items 37–41, 43); and 'supervision' (items 22–26, 29). Total sub-scale score is the sum of all 27 items; because items 29 and 43 are used in more than one of the sub-scales, the total must be computed by adding up the items separately, not just by summing the sub-scale scores (see Chapter 11).

Scoring

Depending on the objectives of the study, the IEQ–EU can be scored in two different ways. For research purposes the five-point Likert scale is recommended. Sub-scale scores based on these categories can be used for the computation of correlations with other instruments. In clinical use average sub-scale scores are not easy to interpret, for instance 'caregiver A has a mean tension score of 8.1 on a range of 0–36'. In such cases it might be better to dichotomise scores to 0 ('never' or 'sometimes') or 1 ('regularly', 'often' or 'always'). The relationship between the Likert scale and the dichotomised scale is therefore as follows:

Likert scale	0	1	2	3	4	5
Dichotomised scale	0	0	1	1	1	1

The ranges of scores for the sub-scales using Likert scale scoring are 0–36 for tension, 0–32 for urging, 0–24 for worrying, 0–24 for supervision and 0–108 for total score; using the dichotomised scale the ranges are tension 0–9, urging 0–8, worrying 0–6, supervision 0–6 and total score 0–27.

The sub-scale score based on the dichotomised item scores directly reflects the number of consequences in this domain that are experienced by the caregiver. In our example this would lead to an interpretation: 'caregiver A at least on a regular basis experiences consequences on two of the nine tension items'. Major changes in consequences can also easily be detected when an item score changes from 0 to 1 or the reverse. Collected data may also be interpreted at item level, for instance if a specific consequence needs to be monitored over time.

Using the IEQ–EU

The IEQ–EU can be completed by any caregiver – not just relatives, but also friends and neighbours. To be able to complete all the items in the questionnaire, the caregiver and patient should have been in contact for at least an hour per week either in person or by telephone during the preceding 4 weeks. Caregivers who have had less than an hour's contact per week should omit items referring to actual help and encouragement (see item 15).

When to use it

The IEQ–EU is suitable for both research and clinical use. Because of its modular structure, users can decide for themselves what information they want to collect. The core module should always be included in full, however, in order to compute sub-scale scores. The scope of this questionnaire is broad: as a research instrument it can be used in large samples to study the relationship between caregiving consequences and population or community characteristics; as a clinical instrument it can used to evaluate the effects of clinical interventions on caregiving consequences.

Conditions for use

There is no charge for use of the IEQ–EU. In order to monitor the use of this instrument and its further development, the authors would like to be kept informed of its use; please contact them before making any translation of the questionnaire.

Applicability

The IEQ–EU is easy to understand and quick to complete: the entire questionnaire takes about 20–30 minutes, and the core module alone about 10 minutes. It can also be administered over the telephone. Its good applicability is demonstrated by high response rates and the high quality of the resulting data. In a study in the Netherlands, 1000 members of an organisation for relatives of people with psychosis were sent the questionnaire by post: the response was 70.2% after two reminders, and of the 702 returned questionnaires only 2 were incomplete (Schene & van Wijngaarden, 1993). In a study of caregivers of people with depression the response rate was 81%, and only 2 out of 262 questionnaires could not be used because of missing data (van Wijngaarden *et al*, 1996). The response rates in the EPSILON Study were not known exactly: the questionnaire was completed and returned on average in 70% of cases; only 9 out of 288 questionnaires could not be used because of missing data (van Wijngaarden *et al*, 2000).

Information

Further information can be obtained from Professor Aart H. Schene, Academic Medical Centre, University of Amsterdam, PO Box 22700, 1100DE Amsterdam, The Netherlands.

References

Beardslee, W. R., Bemporad, J., Keller, M. B., *et al* (1983) Children of parents with major affective disorder; a review. *American Journal of Psychiatry*, **140**, 825–832.

Beisser, A. R., Glaser, N. & Grant, M. (1967) Psychosocial adjustment in children of schizophrenic mothers. *Journal of Nervous and Mental Disorders*, **145**, 429–440.

Biegel, D. E., Sales, E. & Schulz, R. (1991) *Family Caregiving in Chronic Illness*. London: Sage.

Brown, G. W. & Rutter, M. (1966) The measurement of family activities and relationships. *Human Relations*, **19**, 239–263.

Creer, C., Sturt, E. & Wykes, T. (1982) The role of relatives. *Psychological Medicine Monograph Supplement*, **2**, 29–39.

Fadden, G. B. (1984) *The relatives of patients with depressive disorders: a typology of burden and strategies of coping* (thesis). London: Institute of Psychiatry.

Gallop, R., McKeever, P., Mohide, E. A., *et al* (1991) *Family Care and Chronic Illness: The Caregiving Experience*. Toronto: Faculty of Nursing.

Goldberg, D. & Williams, P. (1988) *A User's Guide to the General Health Questionnaire*. Windsor: NFER/Nelson.

Gubman, G. D., Tessler, T. C. & Willis, G. (1987) Living with the mentally ill: factors affecting household complaints. *Schizophrenia Bulletin*, **13**, 727–736.

Joyce, J., Leese, M. & Szmukler, G. (2000) The experience of caregiving inventory: further evidence. *Social Psychiatry and Psychiatric Epidemiology*, **35**, 185–189.

Maurin, I. T. & Barmann, B. (1990) Burden of mental illness on the family: a critical review. *Archives of Psychiatric Nursing*, **4**, 99–107.

Miller, F., Dworkin, J., Ward, M., *et al* (1990) A preliminary study of unresolved grief in families of seriously mentally ill patients. *Hospital and Community Psychiatry*, **41**, 1321–1325.

Platt, S. (1985) Measuring the burden of psychiatric illness on the family: an evaluation of some rating scales. *Psychological Medicine*, **15**, 383–393.

Sainsbury, P. & Grad, J. (1962) Evaluation of treatment and services. In *The Burden on the Community: A Symposium*. London: Oxford University Press.

Schene, A. H. (1986) *Worried at Home: A Monograph on Burden on the Family in Psychiatry* (in Dutch). Utrecht: Netherlands Institute for Mental Health.

Schene, A. H. (1990) Objective and subjective dimensions of family burden: towards an integrative framework for research. *Social Psychiatry and Psychiatric Epidemiology*, **25**, 289–297.

Schene, A. H. & van Wijngaarden, B (1993) *Family Members of People with a Psychotic Disorder: A Study Among Members of Ypsilon* (in Dutch). Amsterdam: Department of Psychiatry, University of Amsterdam.

Szmukler, G. (1996) From family 'burden' to caregiving. *Psychiatric Bulletin*, **20**, 449–451.

Szmukler, G. I., Burgess, P., Herrman, H., *et al* (1996) Caring for relatives with serious mental illness: the development of the experience of caregiving inventory. *Social Psychiatry and Psychiatric Epidemiology*, **31**, 137–148.

Treudley, M. B. (1946) Mental illness and family routines. *Mental Hygiene*, **30**, 235–249.

Van Wijngaarden, B., Schene, A. H. & Koeter, M. W. J. (1996) *The Consequences of Depressive Disorders for Those Involved with the Patient: A Study on the Psychometric Qualities of the Involvement Evaluation Questionnaire* (in Dutch). Amsterdam: Department of Psychiatry, University of Amsterdam.

Van Wijngaarden, B., Schene, A. H., Koeter, M. W. J., *et al* (2000) Caregiving in schizophrenia: development, internal consistency and reliability of the Involvement Evaluation Questionnaire – European Version. The EPSILON Study 4. *British Journal of Psychiatry*, **177**, 21–27.

Van Wijngaarden, B., Schene, A. H., Koeter, M. W. J., *et al* (2003) People with schizophrenia in five countries: conceptual similarities and intercultural differences in family caregiving. *Schizophrenia Bulletin*, **29**, 573–586.

11 Development and reliability of the IEQ–EU

Aart Schene, Bob van Wijngaarden and Maarten Koeter

The development of the IEQ started in 1986 (Schene, 1986). An instrument was needed that could measure caregiving consequences in a randomised controlled trial comparing in-patient and day patient treatment (Schene *et al*, 1993). Since no such instrument existed at that time in the Netherlands, we developed one ourselves, starting with an extensive review of all empirical studies on family burden over the preceding 40 years (Schene, 1986; Schene *et al*, 1994). An item pool was created drawn from the literature and from existing research instruments (Schene *et al*, 1994, 1996), such as the Family Distress Scale (Pasamanick *et al*, 1967), the Family Evaluation Form (Spitzer *et al*, 1971), the Family Burden Scale (Test & Stein, 1980) and the Family Distress Scale for Depression (Jacob *et al*, 1987). This item pool was further extended with items emerging from interviews with professionals.

Next, the desirable characteristics for such a research instrument were defined: it should be a self-administered questionnaire, short but comprehensive, and covering a limited time frame; it should be sensitive to change and should focus on the more objective consequences of caregiving. It should enable assessment of exactly what caregiving implies in terms of tasks, costs, time consumption and frequency. A series of draft versions were piloted and adapted. Since the principal aim was to develop a reliable measure that would be sensitive to change, items relating to stigma, guilt and social network loss were dropped, along with items about other events that either happen rarely or are insensitive to change, such as suicide attempts.

Initially it was considered important that the person filling out the questionnaire should be someone who lived in the same household as the patient. Items were formulated accordingly, speaking of 'the ill member of your household' instead of 'your ill relative'. This made the questionnaire also suitable for those who shared households with the patient but who were not relatives. As the main objective was to assess the objective aspects of caregiving, the questions were formulated in such a way that they referred to the frequency of occurrence of a particular event (for instance, a quarrel between the relative and the patient), and not how burdensome this event was for the relative.

The first version of the instrument, the Burden on the Family scale (BoF; Schene, 1987) was produced in 1987 and tested in four Dutch studies conducted between 1987 and 1990: (a) a comparative study of day treatment *v*. in-patient treatment (*n*=80; Schene *et al*, 1993); (b) a study of caregivers of patients who had recently attempted suicide (*n*=80); (c) a study in the psychiatric department of a general hospital (*n*=80); and (d) a study of acute psychiatric patients in a community mental health centre (*n*=30). These studies revealed that this instrument's focus on household members restricted its use: no information could be obtained about the many patients who lived alone but who were in contact with caregivers. To solve this problem, we decided to widen the scope of the instrument to all caregivers.

Research on the BoF resulted in a series of adaptations. Major changes concerned the wording of items, the deletion of 'bad' items and the addition of items that emerged from an updated review of the literature from 1986 to 1991, in particular with regard to depression and caregiving. We added, for example, a series of items concerning caregiver's worrying, a set of demographic variables and items regarding the relationship between relative and patient, household composition, and duration of illness. In 1992 these adaptations finally resulted in the Betrokkenen Evaluatie Schaal (BES), translated into English as the Involvement Evaluation Questionnaire (Schene & van Wijngaarden, 1992a,b).

Translations

Since the 1992 English translation the IEQ has been translated into Finnish, French, German, Portuguese and Swedish. In 1997 the IEQ was chosen to be one of the core instruments in the EPSILON Study for development into a standardised version with cross-cultural validity and reliability (Becker *et al*, 1999). The translation of the IEQ into Danish, Italian and Spanish for the EPSILON Study largely followed the protocol described in Chapter 2, and resulted in a standardised European version in these languages, now labelled as the IEQ–EU.

Scale structure

The scale structure of the 1992 version of the IEQ was tested in two Dutch studies, one among 680 members of an organisation of relatives of patients with psychotic disorders (Schene & van Wijngaarden, 1993, 1995), and one among 260 relatives of patients with affective disorders (van Wijngaarden *et al*, 1996). Separate principal component analyses on both samples led to very comparable factor solutions, and in both samples the items loaded on the same factors. This finding indicated a common underlying factor structure, which was confirmed by simultaneous components analysis (Kiers, 1990). This meant that the IEQ adequately covered all major domains of caregiving consequences for both relatives of people with psychosis and caregivers of people with depressive disorder (van Wijngaarden *et al*, 1996). The next step was finding a scale structure that would fit both samples best.

Factor analysis on the core module items of the combined sample (*n*=940) resulted in a four-factor solution, which accounted for 59.6% of the total variance. Of the 28 items that were entered in this analysis, 25 loaded more than 0.40 on one of the factors. Only item 36 ('able to pursue own activities') had loadings lower than 0.40, and so this item was omitted from the scale. The four factors and the total score can be summarised as follows:

- *Tension* refers to the strained interpersonal atmosphere between patient and relatives and/or caregivers (nine items: 29–35, 42, 43; scale score 0–36);
- *Urging* refers to activation and motivations, such as stimulating the patient to take care of him- or herself, to eat enough and to undertake activities (eight items: 16–21, 27, 28; scale score 0–32);
- *Worrying* covers painful interpersonal cognitions, such as concern about the patient's safety and future, general health and health care (six items: 37–41, 43; scale score 0–24);
- *Supervision* refers to the caregiver's tasks of guarding the patient's medicine intake, sleep and dangerous behaviour (six items: 22–26, 29; scale score 0–24);
- *Total score* is the sum of all 27 items; because items 29 and 43 are used in more than one scale, the total score must be computed by adding up the 27 items separately and not by just adding up the four sub-scales (scores 0–108).

Validity

The validity of the IEQ was studied in the two samples that were also used in the factor analysis. The content validity proved to be satisfactory. The validity of the 1992 version of the instrument was confirmed by a qualitative analysis of item 81, an open question asking respondents to add any issue that bothered, stressed or satisfied them in their relationship to the patient, and that was not covered by the IEQ. Although many caregivers used this question to express their caregiving experiences, the analysis of 680 questionnaires did not reveal any missing domains or variables (Schene & van Wijngaarden, 1993). Finally, the fact that separate analyses of the data regarding relatives of psychotic or depressed patients revealed factor structures that were very comparable with those of the combined sample can also be considered as an indicator of content validity.

Construct validity could not be assessed properly because there was no other Dutch research measure of caregiver consequences that could be used as an external criterion. However, circumstantial evidence for satisfactory construct validity was found. The conceptual models presented in this chapter predicted a major role for patient's symptoms and symptom behaviour as independent variables, and variables such as caregiver's coping style, social support and mental health care system charactistics as mediators (Biegel *et al*, 1991; Gallop *et al*, 1991; Maurin & Barmann, 1990; Schene, 1990; Szmukler *et al*, 1996). In both Dutch studies proofs for these models were found. In accordance with the models, high IEQ scores could be predicted from the severity of the patient's symptoms, deterioration of the illness since onset, less caregiver's coping ability, more caregiver contacts with mental health professionals, and more time spent with the patient, in the sample of relatives of people with psychotic disorders. Explained variances ranged from 21% for 'urging' to 55% for 'tension'. Also, a high correlation of 0.50 was found between the IEQ and caregiver distress scores (Schene & van Wijngaarden, 1993).

In a sample of caregivers of people with depression, comparable correlations were found. High IEQ scores could be predicted by a high level of patient symptoms, inadequate coping strategies, lack of social support, and more time spent with the patient. Moreover, caregivers of people whose depression was still florid had higher IEQ scores than caregivers of people whose condition had stabilised with medication. Although correlations were not as strong as in the other sample (explained variances ranged from 0.20 to 0.42), these finding matched the results from the first study (van Wijngaarden *et al*, 1996). Path analysis on the first data-set showed that the caregiving consequences measured with the IEQ explained a substantial part of the relation between the caregiver's distress and the patient, caregiver and relationship characteristics (Schene *et al*, 1998). This finding corresponds with the distinction made between objective and subjective caregiving consequences. As we saw in the other analyses, the 'objective' IEQ scores reflect things that the caregiver has to do as a result of the patients's illness. The path analysis showed caregiving to be a precursor of subjective consequences (i.e. caregiver distress), which emphasises the conceptual relevance of the IEQ.

The validity of the IEQ–EU translations proved to be good. The uniform, standardised and well-documented protocol, following World Health Organization regulations, ensured high-quality translations (see Chapter 2). In all focus group meetings it was concluded that the items of the IEQ were clear, that they covered the relevant domains of caregiver consequences, and that no important issue was missing (Knudsen *et al*, 2000).

Concept validity also proved to be good. First, validity was tested by comparing the patterns of the mean IEQ item scores between the five countries. These patterns were almost identical, and they also matched the patterns found in the original Dutch studies. This means that in all countries, worrying about the patient's health, future, safety and financial position were the most frequently mentioned caregiving consequences, followed by the necessity to urge the patient to do something. Also in all countries, need for supervision and interpersonal tension were the consequences mentioned least. Second, concept validity was tested by means of simultaneous components analysis (SCA; Kiers, 1990), an analysis that finds the best factor solution for more than one data-set simultaneously, where the joint factor solution reflects the optimium fit for each of these data-sets. The SCA factor solution proved to be very similar to the original Dutch factors, meaning that the underlying structure of the IEQ is invariant over all sites (van Wijngaarden *et al*, 2003).

Reliability

The reliability of the IEQ proved to be satisfactory in the Dutch samples. The internal consistency (Cronbach's α) ranged from 0.74 to 0.85 for the four sub-scales and was 0.90 for the total scores. Test–retest effects were not found, and the IEQ proved to be sensitive to change (van Wijngaarden *et al*, 1996; Stam & Cuijpers, 1999). In the EPSILON project reliability testing was one of the main objectives (Becker *et al*, 1999). Reliability was tested in two ways:

(a) internal consistency: Cronbach's alphas were computed for each site separately and inter-site differences were tested;
(b) test–retest reliability: intraclass correlation coefficients (ICCs) were computed and inter-site differences tested.

Benchmarks were set to 0.70 for substantial reliability and 0.80 for high reliability. For more details on the reliability methodology, see Chapter 3.

Cronbach's alpha and ICC values are presented in Table 11.1. The shaded areas represent reliability values that did not reach one or both benchmarks. The alpha values ranged from 0.68 to 0.91. In 20 out of 30 cases (67%), reliability was high. However, in two cases – 'supervision' in London and 'urging' in Santander – the benchmark for substantial reliability was just not reached, both having a value of 0.68. Alpha testing between sites revealed that only on the sub-scale 'urging' were differences significant. Alpha in Santander was lowest (0.68), that in London was highest (0.86). In all but one case ('worrying' in Verona), test–retest reliability was substantial to high, with a range of 0.70 to 0.99. Intraclass correlation coefficients proved to be highest in Amsterdam, Copenhagen and London, demonstrating good reliability. Although all reliabilities are substantial, in Santander the ICCs for

Table 11.1 Internal consistency (α) and test–retest reliability (ICC) of the Involvement Evaluation Questionnaire in the five EPSILON sites

Sub-scale	Pooled n=335 α ICC	Amsterdam n=88 α ICC	Copenhagen n=30 α ICC	London n=75 α ICC	Santander n=78 α ICC	Verona n=64 α ICC	α equality test P	ICC equality test P
Tension	0.81	0.78	0.75	0.80	0.80	0.84	0.58	
	0.89	0.92	0.95	0.97	0.82	0.88		<0.01
Worrying	0.84	0.86	0.84	0.77	0.83	0.82	0.55	
	0.84	0.87	0.93	0.98	0.78	0.69		<0.01
Urging	0.79	0.82	0.71	0.86	0.68	0.81	0.03[1]	
	0.89	0.93	0.80	0.98	0.73	0.90		<0.01
Supervision	0.77	0.80	0.73	0.68	0.75	0.82	0.47	
	0.83	0.87	0.98	0.97	0.70	0.82		<0.01
Total score	0.90	0.91	0.87	0.89	0.87	0.91	0.45	
	0.90	0.94	0.93	0.99	0.81	0.86		<0.01

1. Differences were found between: Amsterdam–Santander *P*<0.001; London–Santander *P*<0.001; London–Copenhagen *P*<0.05; Santander–Verona *P*<0.05.

supervision, worrying and urging are somewhat lower than the sometimes very high values in the other sites. In none of the cases were both internal consistency and test reliability below benchmark values.

In summary, it can be concluded that the IEQ scales have substantial to high reliability in all sites (van Wijngaarden *et al*, 2000). Combined with the good applicability and the satisfactory to good validity, the IEQ proves to be a useful instrument for the assessment of caregiving consequences in at least five European countries.

References and further reading

Becker, T., Knapp, M., Knudsen, H. C., *et al* (1999) The EPSILON study of schizophrenia in five European countries: design and methodology for standardising outcome measures and comparing patterns of care and service costs. *British Journal of Psychiatry*, **175**, 514–521.

Becker, T., Knapp, M., Knudsen, H. C., *et al* (2000) Aims, outcome measures, study sites and patient sample. EPSILON Study 1. *British Journal of Psychiatry*, **177** (suppl. 39), s1–s7.

Biegel, D. E., Sales, E. & Schulz, R. (1991) *Family Caregiving in Chronic Illness*. London: Sage.

Gallop, R., McKeever, P., Mohide, E. A., *et al* (1991) *Family Care and Chronic Illness: The Caregiving Experience. A Review of the Literature*. Toronto: Faculty of Nursing.

Jacob, M., Frank, E., Kupfer, D. J., *et al* (1987) Recurrent depression: an assessment of family burden and family attitudes. *Journal of Clinical Psychiatry*, **48**, 395–400.

Kiers, H. A. L. (1990) *SCA: A Program for Simultaneous Components Analysis of Variables Measured in Two or More Populations*. Groningen: iec ProGAMMA.

Knudsen, H. C., Vázquez-Barquero, J. L., Welcher, B., *et al* (2000) Translation and cross-cultural adaptation of outcome measurements for schizophrenia. EPSILON Study 2. *British Journal of Psychiatry*, **177** (suppl. 39), s8–s14.

Maurin, I. T. & Barmann, B. (1990) Burden of mental illness on the family: a critical review. *Archives of Psychiatric Nursing*, **4**, 99–107.

Pasamanick, B., Scarpitti, F. R. & Dinitz, S. (1967) *Schizophrenics in the Community: An Experimental Study in the Prevention of Hospitalization*. New York: Appleton-Century-Crofts.

Schene, A. H. (1986) *Worried at Home; A Monograph on Burden on the Family in Psychiatry* [in Dutch]. Utrecht: Nederlands Centrum Geestelijke Volksgezondheid (Netherlands Institute for Mental Health).

Schene, A. H. (1987) *De Burden On the Family Schaal (BOF): A Questionnaire for the Assessment of Burden for Relatives of Psychiatric Patients* [in Dutch]. Utrecht: Department of Psychiatry, University of Amsterdam.

Schene, A. H. (1990) Objective and subjective dimensions of family burden: towards an integrative framework for research. *Social Psychiatry and Psychiatric Epidemiology*, **25**, 289–297.

Schene, A. H. & van Wijngaarden, B. (1992a) *De Betrokkenen Evaluatie Schaal (BES)* [in Dutch]. Amsterdam: Department of Psychiatry, University of Amsterdam.

Schene, A. H. & van Wijngaarden, B. (1992b) *The Involvement Evaluation Questionnaire*. Amsterdam: Department of Psychiatry, University of Amsterdam.

Schene, A. H. & van Wijngaarden, B. (1993) *Family Members of People with a Psychotic Disorder: A Study Among Members of Ypsilon* [in Dutch]. Amsterdam: Department of Psychiatry, University of Amsterdam.

Schene, A. H. & van Wijngaarden, B. (1995) A survey of an organization for families of patients with serious mental illness in the Netherlands. *Psychiatric Services*, **46**, 807–813.

Schene, A., van Wijngaarden, B, Poelijoe, N. W., *et al* (1993) The Utrecht comparative study on psychiatric day treatment and inpatient treatment. *Acta Psychiatrica Scandinavica*, **87**, 427–436.

Schene, A. H., Tessler, R. C. & Gamache, G. M. (1994) Instruments measuring family or caregiver burden in severe mental illness. *Social Psychiatry and Psychiatric Epidemiology*, **29**, 228–240.

Schene, A. H., Tessler, R. C. & Gamache, G. M. (1996) Caregiving in severe mental illness: conceptualization and measurement. In *Mental Health Service Evaluation* (eds H. C. Knudsen & G. Thornicroft), pp. 296–316. Cambridge: Cambridge University Press.

Schene, A. H., van Wijngaarden, B. & Koeter, M. W. J. (1998) Family caregiving in schizophrenia: domains and distress. *Schizophrenia Bulletin*, **24**, 609–618.

Spitzer, R. L., Giboon, M. & Endicott, J. (1971) *Family Evaluation Form*. New York: New York State Department of Mental Hygiene.

Stam, H. & Cuijpers, P. (1999) *Psycho-Education for Relatives of Psychiatric Patients: The Effects on Burden* [in Dutch]. Utrecht: Netherlands Institute of Mental Health and Addiction.

Szmukler, G. I., Burgess, P., Herrman, H., *et al* (1996) Caring for relatives with serious mental illness: the development of the Experience of Caregiving Inventory. *Social Psychiatry and Psychiatric Epidemiology*, **31**, 137–148.

Test, M. A. & Stein, L. I. (1980) Alternative to mental hospital treatment. III: Social cost. *Archives of General Psychiatry*, **37**, 409–412.

van Wijngaarden, B., Schene, A. H. & Koeter, M. W. J. (1996) *The Consequences of Depressive Disorders for Those Involved with the Patient: A Study on the Psychometric Qualities of the Involvement Evaluation Questionnaire* ([n Dutch]. Amsterdam: Department of Psychiatry, University of Amsterdam.

Van Wijngaarden, B., Schene, A. H., Koeter, M. W. J., *et al* (2000) Caregiving in schizophrenia: development, internal consistency and reliability of the Involvement Evaluation Questionnaire – European Version. The EPSILON Study 4. *British Journal of Psychiatry*, **177**, 21–27.

Van Wijngaarden, B., Schene, A. H., Koeter, M. W. J., *et al* (2003) People with schizophrenia in five countries: conceptual similarities and intercultural differences in family caregiving. *Schizophrenia Bulletin*, **29**, 573–586.

Vázquez-Barquero, J. L. & García, J. (1999) Deinstitutionalization and psychiatric reform in Spain. *European Archives of Psychiatry and Clinical Neuroscience*, **249**, 120–135.

Wing, J. K., Monck, E., Brown, G. W., *et al* (1959) Morbidity in the community of schizophrenic patients discharged from London mental hospitals in 1959. *British Journal of Psychiatry*, **110**, 10–21.

12 Involvement Evaluation Questionnaire – European Version

Aart Schene, Bob van Wijngaarden and Maarten Koeter

In the field of psychiatric care, attention has been concentrated almost exclusively on the patients themselves. In recent years, however, more concern has been shown towards the families, friends and others involved.

You too are involved in the care of someone with mental health problems and this questionnaire has been designed to assess the personal consequences of such a situation for carers like yourself.

Completing the questionnaire

The questionnaire is divided into eight sections, each representing a different aspect of caring. Each part is headed by a brief explanatory paragraph to lead you into the theme of the section.

Only **one answer** is possible for each question, unless otherwise indicated – please tick accordingly. In some cases, we will ask you to fill in a few personal details, such as your age.

It is quite possible that in some cases, a question will not be relevant to your particular circumstances. The questionnaire will clearly indicate, therefore, which questions you can ignore and at which point you should start again.

The consequences of your caring for someone who has mental health problems might have existed for several years already, but it is important to bear in mind that this questionnaire is mostly concerned with an analysis of the **current situation**. Most of the questions, therefore, cover your experiences over the **past 4 weeks**, while a few questions are about your more long-term experience. The questions themselves will make this clear.

All information will be treated confidentially, and you do not have to give your name if you do not wish to. If there are questions that you would prefer not to answer, we will, of course, respect your wishes – in this case, however, please write '**no answer**' next to the question.

Take your time to answer each question in turn and remember that what matters most of all is that your answers truly reflect your own personal experience.

Involvement Evaluation Questionnaire – European Version

General information

Today's date (DD/MM/YY) ▢▢/▢▢/▢▢

Before we turn to the matter of your own experiences, we would first like to have some general information about you personally and about the relative/friend you are caring for.

1. What is your age?   Years: ▢▢

2. What is your gender?   ▢ Male
                                          ▢ Female

3. Please describe your education
    and training: _____
                                          _____
                                          _____
                                          _____

4. What is your civil status?   ▢ Single
                                          ▢ Married/in a long-term partnership
                                          ▢ Divorced
                                          ▢ Widowed

5. Do you live alone or with others?   ▢ I live alone (**proceed to question 7**)
                                          ▢ I live with my spouse/partner and/or children
                                          ▢ I live with my parents and/or sisters/brothers
                                          ▢ I live with other relatives
                                          ▢ I live with friends
                                          ▢ Other _____

6. How many people, including yourself,
    are there in your household?   Number of people: ▢▢

7. What is the age of your relative/friend?   Years: ▢▢

8. What is the gender of your relative/friend?   ▢ Male
                                                  ▢ Female

9. When did your relative/friend's mental
    health problems start?   Year: ▢▢▢▢

10. Is your relative/friend currently receiving help for his/her mental health problems?
    (Please note that more than one answer is possible)

    ☐ I do not know

    ☐ No professional help

    ☐ Yes, from a GP/family doctor

    ☐ Yes, from a social worker

    ☐ Yes, from an occupational therapist

    ☐ Yes, at the community mental health centre/from the community mental health team

    ☐ Yes, from a psychologist or cognitive–behavioural therapist

    ☐ Yes, as an out-patient at a psychiatric hospital or the psychiatric department of a general hospital

    ☐ Yes, in a psychiatric day hospital

    ☐ Yes, as an in-patient in a psychiatric hospital or the psychiatric department of a general hospital

    ☐ Yes, living in supported housing

    ☐ Yes, other (please specify)

11. What is your precise relationship with your relative/friend?
    I am his/her:

    ☐ Mother/father (step, foster and adoptive parents included)

    ☐ Daughter/son

    ☐ Sister/brother

    ☐ Other relative

    ☐ Spouse, partner or girl/boyfriend

    ☐ Friend

    ☐ Neighbour

    ☐ Colleague/fellow student

    ☐ Other _____

12. Is you relative/friend part of your household?   ☐ Yes
                                                       ☐ No

13. How many days have you and your relative/friend lived together at the same address during the past 4 weeks?

    ☐ None

    ☐ Some days. How many? ☐☐

    ☐ The full 4 weeks

14. What is your family's approximate *net* income (wage/salary, welfare benefits, pension, etc., after deductions for tax, National Insurance, etc.)

☐ Less than £300 per month   (less than €500 per month)

☐ £300–£500 per month   (€500–800 per month)

☐ £500–£900 per month   (€800–1400 per month)

☐ £900–£1500 per month   (€1400–2400 per month)

☐ £1500–£2250 per month   (€2400–3500 per month)

☐ More than £2250 per month   (more than €3500 per month)

15. What has been your average *weekly* telephone or personal contact with your relative/friend over the past 4 weeks?

☐ Less than 1 hour per week **(proceed to Question 37)**

☐ 1–4 hours a week

☐ 5–8 hours a week

☐ 9–16 hours a week

☐ 17–32 hours a week

☐ More than 32 hours a week

The following questions are about the encouragement and care you have given to your relative/friend over the past 4 weeks

16. How often during the past 4 weeks have you **encouraged** your relative/friend to take proper care of her/himself (e.g. washing, bathing, brushing teeth, dressing, combing hair, etc.)?

☐ Never

☐ Sometimes

☐ Regularly

☐ Often

☐ (almost) Always

17. How often during the past 4 weeks have you **helped** your relative/friend take proper care of him/herself (e.g. washing, bathing, brushing teeth, dressing, combing hair, etc.)?

☐ Never

☐ Sometimes

☐ Regularly

☐ Often

☐ (almost) Always

18. How often during the past 4 weeks have you **encouraged** your relative/friend to eat enough?

    ☐ Never
    ☐ Sometimes
    ☐ Regularly
    ☐ Often
    ☐ (almost) Always

19. How often over the past 4 weeks have you **encouraged** your relative/friend to undertake some kind of activity (e.g. go for a walk, have a chat, hobbies, household chores)?

    ☐ Never
    ☐ Sometimes
    ☐ Regularly
    ☐ Often
    ☐ (almost) Always

20. How often during the past 4 weeks have you **accompanied** your relative/friend on some kind of outside activity, because he/she did not dare to go alone?

    ☐ Never
    ☐ Sometimes
    ☐ Regularly
    ☐ Often
    ☐ (almost) Always

21. How often during the past 4 weeks have you **ensured** that your relative/friend has taken the required medicine?

    ☐ Not relevant: relative/friend has no medicines
    ☐ Never
    ☐ Sometimes
    ☐ Regularly
    ☐ Often
    ☐ (almost) Always)

22. How often during the past 4 weeks have you **guarded** your relative/friend from committing dangerous acts (i.e. setting something alight, leaving the gas on, forgetting to stub cigarettes out, etc.)?

    ☐ Never

    ☐ Sometimes

    ☐ Regularly

    ☐ Often

    ☐ (almost) Always

23. How often during the past 4 weeks have you **guarded** your relative/friend from self-inflicted harm (i.e. cutting him/herself, excessive medication intake, burning, suicide attempt, etc.)?

    ☐ Never

    ☐ Sometimes

    ☐ Regularly

    ☐ Often

    ☐ (almost) Always

24. How often during the past 4 weeks have you **ensured** that your relative/friend received sufficient sleep?

    ☐ Never

    ☐ Sometimes

    ☐ Regularly

    ☐ Often

    ☐ (almost) Always

25. How often during the past 4 weeks have you **guarded** your relative/friend from drinking too much alcohol?

    ☐ Never

    ☐ Sometimes

    ☐ Regularly

    ☐ Often

    ☐ (almost) Always

26. How often during the past 4 weeks have you **guarded** your relative/friend from taking illegal drugs?

    ☐ Never

    ☐ Sometimes

    ☐ Regularly

    ☐ Often

    ☐ (almost) Always

27. How often during the past 4 weeks have you **carried out** tasks normally done by your relative/friend (household chores, financial matters, shopping, cooking, etc.)?

    ☐ Never

    ☐ Sometimes

    ☐ Regularly

    ☐ Often

    ☐ (almost) Always

28. How often during the past 4 weeks have you **encouraged** your relative/friend to get up in the morning?

    ☐ Never

    ☐ Sometimes

    ☐ Regularly

    ☐ Often

    ☐ (almost) Always

29. How often during the past 4 weeks has your relative/friend disturbed your sleep?

    ☐ Never

    ☐ Sometimes

    ☐ Regularly

    ☐ Often

    ☐ (almost) Always

> *The following questions are about how you have got on with your relative/friend in the past 4 weeks.*

30. How often during the past 4 weeks has the atmosphere been strained between you both, as a result of your relative/friend's behaviour?

    ☐ Never
    ☐ Sometimes
    ☐ Regularly
    ☐ Often
    ☐ (almost) Always

31. How often during the past 4 weeks has your relative/friend caused a quarrel?

    ☐ Never
    ☐ Sometimes
    ☐ Regularly
    ☐ Often
    ☐ (almost) Always

32. How often during the past 4 weeks have you been annoyed by your relative/friend's behaviour?

    ☐ Never
    ☐ Sometimes
    ☐ Regularly
    ☐ Often
    ☐ (almost) Always

33. How often during the past 4 weeks have you heard from **others** that they have been annoyed by your relative/friend's behaviour?

    ☐ Never
    ☐ Sometimes
    ☐ Regularly
    ☐ Often
    ☐ (almost) Always

34. How often during the past 4 weeks have you felt threatened by your relative/friend?

    ☐ Never

    ☐ Sometimes

    ☐ Regularly

    ☐ Often

    ☐ (almost) Always

35. How often during the past 4 weeks have you thought of moving out, as a result of your relative/friend's behaviour?

    ☐ Never

    ☐ Sometimes

    ☐ Regularly

    ☐ Often

    ☐ (almost) Always

36. How often during the past 4 weeks have you been able to pursue your own activities and interests (e.g. work, school, hobbies, sports, visits to family and friends)?

    ☐ Never

    ☐ Sometimes

    ☐ Regularly

    ☐ Often

    ☐ (almost) Always

The following questions are about the worries that may arise from your involvement with a relative/friend who has mental health problems.

37. How often during the past 4 weeks have you **worried** about your relative/friend's **safety?**

    ☐ Never

    ☐ Sometimes

    ☐ Regularly

    ☐ Often

    ☐ (almost) Always

38. How often during the past 4 weeks have you **worried** about the kind of **help/treatment** your relative/friend is receiving?

- [ ] Never
- [ ] Sometimes
- [ ] Regularly
- [ ] Often
- [ ] (almost) Always

39. How often during the past 4 weeks have you **worried** about your relative/friend's **general health?**

- [ ] Never
- [ ] Sometimes
- [ ] Regularly
- [ ] Often
- [ ] (almost) Always

40. How often during the past 4 weeks have you **worried** about how your relative/friend would manage financially if you were no longer able to help?

- [ ] Never
- [ ] Sometimes
- [ ] Regularly
- [ ] Often
- [ ] (almost) Always

41. How often during the past 4 weeks have you **worried** about your relative/friend's **future?**

- [ ] Never
- [ ] Sometimes
- [ ] Regularly
- [ ] Often
- [ ] (almost) Always

42. How often during the past 4 weeks have you **worried** about **your own future?**

- [ ] Never
- [ ] Sometimes
- [ ] Regularly
- [ ] Often
- [ ] (almost) Always

43. To what extent have your relative/friend's mental health problems been a **burden** to you during the past 4 weeks?

☐ No burden at all
☐ A slight burden
☐ A fairly heavy burden
☐ A heavy burden
☐ A very heavy burden

44. Have you got used to your relative/friend having mental health problems?

☐ No
☐ A little
☐ Fairly well
☐ Very well
☐ Completely

45. How often have you felt able to cope with your relative/friend's mental health problems?

☐ Never
☐ Sometimes
☐ Regularly
☐ Often
☐ (almost) Always

46. Has your relationship with your relative/friend changed **since the onset** of the mental health problems?

☐ No
☐ A little
☐ Rather a lot
☐ A lot
☐ A great deal

The following questions are about the financial cost to you and your household, as a result of your relative/friend's mental health problems.

Have you, during the past 4 weeks, had to incur extra expenses **on behalf of your relative/friend?**

	Yes	No
47. Professional help for your relative/friend	☐	☐
48. Damage caused by your relative/friend	☐	☐
49. Large expenditures incurred by your relative/friend	☐	☐
50. Relative/friend's travel expenses	☐	☐
51. Medicine for your relative/friend	☐	☐
52. Paying off debts incurred by your relative/friend	☐	☐

53. Other expenses (please indicate) _____

54. If you add up all the **extra expenses** that you have incurred on behalf of your relative/friend **during the past 4 weeks**, what is the estimated total figure?

☐ Less than £25 (less than €50)
☐ £25–£50 (€50–80)
☐ £50–£125 (€80–200)
☐ £125–£250 (€200–400)
☐ More than £250 (more than €400)

*Please read the questions below and each of the four possible answers. We want to know how your health has been in general over the **past four weeks**. Please answer **all** the questions by circling the response that best applies to you.*

Have you recently:

55. been able to concentrate on what you are doing?	Better than usual	Same as usual	Less than usual	Much less than usual
56. lost much sleep over worry?	Not at all	No more than usual	Rather more than usual	Much more than usual
57. felt that you are playing a useful part in things?	More so than usual	Same as usual	Less so than usual	Much less than usual
58. felt capable of making decisions about things?	More so than usual	Same as usual	Less so than usual	Much less capable
59. felt constantly under strain?	Not at all	No more than usual	Rather more than usual	Much more than usual

60. felt you couldn't overcome your difficulties?	Not at all	No more than usual	Rather more than usual	Much more than usual
61. been able to enjoy normal day-to-day activities?	More so than usual	Same as usual	Less so than usual	Much less than usual
62. been able to face up to your problems?	More so than usual	Same as usual	Less able than usual	Much less able
63. been feeling unhappy or depressed?	Not at all	No more than usual	Rather more than usual	Much more than usual
64. been losing confidence in yourself?	Not at all	No more than usual	Rather more than usual	Much more than usual
65. been thinking of yourself as a worthless person?	Not at all	No more than usual	Rather more than usual	Much more than usual
66. been feeling reasonably happy, all things considered	More so than usual	Same as usual	Less so than usual	Much less than usual

67. Are you receiving help from your GP/family doctor for any of these complaints?

☐ Yes
☐ No

68. Are you receiving help from a social worker, a psychologist, a psychiatrist or an out-patient department for any of these complaints?

☐ Yes
☐ No

69. Are you taking any kind of medicine for these complaints?

☐ Yes
☐ No

If a father or mother has mental health problems, this may have consequences for their children, if any. The following questions are about these consequences.

70. Has your relative/friend with mental health problems any children (including step/foster/adopted children)?

☐ No (**proceed to question 81**)
☐ Yes (number of children: ___)

71. Has your relative/friend any children under the age of 16 years?

☐ No (**proceed to question 81**)
☐ Yes (number under 16: ___)

How often has it happened in the past 4 weeks that the child/children has/have:

	Never	Sometimes	Often	Don't know
72. Shown loss of appetite	☐	☐	☐	☐
73. Been sleepless at night	☐	☐	☐	☐
74. Been less attentive at school	☐	☐	☐	☐
75. Shown fear of father/mother	☐	☐	☐	☐
76. Not attended school	☐	☐	☐	☐
77. Displayed difficult behaviour	☐	☐	☐	☐
78. Played less often with friends	☐	☐	☐	☐
79. Felt ashamed of mother/father	☐	☐	☐	☐
80. Had to stay with neighbours, relatives or friends	☐	☐	☐	☐

81. The items listed in this questionnaire cannot, of course, cover all your experiences. If you would like to make any further comments, please feel free to write them in the space below.

Comments

It is important for the purposes of this study that **all the questions that apply to you personally have been answered.**

We would appreciate it, therefore, if you would carefully check that no question has been overlooked.

Please accept our sincere thanks for your help and cooperation.

Part V

Lancashire Quality of Life Profile – European Version

13 Introduction and manual for the LQoLP–EU

Luis Gaite, José Luis Vázquez-Barquero, Jo Oliver and Peter Huxley

The Lancashire Quality of Life Profile (LQoLP) is a structured interview for measuring the health and welfare of people with mental health disorders, particularly those with long-standing, complex and serious conditions. It was based upon American and British research questionnaires developed for use with people with similar life predicaments; to this, original material was added together with questions derived from sources not previously used in this type of research. The interview was piloted in the north-west of England and subsequently used in the UK and elsewhere. The European version (LQoLP–EU) was developed in the context of the EPSILON Study (see Chapter 1).

The LQoLP–EU gives a comprehensive, albeit brief, outline of an individual's current level of psychosocial functioning. It combines objective, factual material related to several different life areas or domains with subjective material drawn from the individual's self-assessment. Also included is a professional assessment of quality of life based on observation and prior knowledge of the case. The interview is intended to strike a balance between the structure required to produce reliable results and the flexibility necessary to create an atmosphere in which the client can feel comfortable discussing personal matters. Continual pruning of the questions has reduced the length of the interview to the minimum necessary to generate a useful profile. The psychometric properties of the LQoLP were verified in the EPSILON Study with good results (see Chapter 14).

Rating instructions

General instructions

The questionnaire should whenever possible be completed in a single interview; experience leads us to believe that an hour is generally sufficient. Only one questionnaire is to be completed for each individual. If for some reason more than one session is required, the same form should be used, continuing from the point at which the previous interview stopped. The interview is best conducted in a quiet place with sufficient privacy to allow the person interviewed to feel able to speak freely without being overheard. As the interview requires the close attention of both people involved, an environment free from interruptions is also desirable.

Information should be gathered in the order it appears on the questionnaire. Answers must be made in the spaces available on the form; scores are entered in the boxes on the right-hand side of each page. All questions must be completed.

Specific instructions

Before beginning the interview it is necessary to introduce oneself, explain to the client the exact purpose of the interview, and gain the client's consent. The following is an example of an introduction that we have found to work well in practice:

'Thank you for allowing me to speak with you. My name is ... and I work for the ... department.' [Social services identification may be displayed at this point if required.] 'I am visiting you because we are interested in finding out all about the things that go to make up your everyday life and how you feel about them. We want to get a fairly complete picture of the quality of your life at present so that we have a better idea of how to develop our services in the future. To do this, I will need to ask you questions about many different areas of living. I expect that I shall take about an hour of your time.

'Before we begin, I should like to say that anything you say to me will be held in confidence. Normally this would mean that only I and my superiors in the department would have access to it and no information will be passed on to others without your knowledge and consent. I hope that this will help you to feel that you can speak openly and honestly with me. Also, you may find some of the questions difficult or too personal to discuss. In either instance, please do not hesitate to say so. You may decline to answer any question you choose, and may also stop the interview at any time. I will certainly understand.'

Initial information

- Name or identifier: affix the client's name or other personal identifier such an identification number. This is necessary to ensure that the same person has not been interviewed twice, and that should the client be contacted again at a later date the information can be accurately updated.
- Interviewer's code: state the interviewer's code for each interview.
- Centre code: state centre's code.
- Date of interview: in the rare event that the questionnaire is completed in two separate interviews, include only the first date.
- Client declines interview: if the client declines to be interviewed, please state the reason if one has been given. Also include here other reasons for not completing the interview, such as acute illness, or the interviewer's opinion that proceeding would not be in the client's best interest. In all circumstances give a clear reason for not proceeding.
- Starting time: be sure to note the time at which the interview actually begins. Comparison with the finishing time allows the length of the interview to be estimated.

Section 1: Client's personal details

1.1   Insert current age to the nearest year.

1.2   Insert the code number for gender, as given in the question.

1.3   Insert the code letter for the ethnic group.

1.4   Insert age of cessation of formal education to nearest year.

If a client is unwilling or unable to answer a question, please insert code 3; if the question is for some reason not applicable to the client, insert code 8 (not applicable).

Section 2: General well-being

Give the client a copy of the Life Satisfaction Scale (LSS), which should be kept by the client for use throughout the interview. This scale helps clients give verbal expression to a range of levels of satisfaction from 'low' ('can't be worse') to 'high' ('can't be better'), and contains a variety of expressions between these two extremes (see page 138). These levels are numbered from 1 (low) to 7 (high). Please record only the number corresponding to the words chosen by the client. The use of the scale may be explained to the client as follows:

> 'Please look at this.' [Show the client the Life Satisfaction Scale.] 'This is a chart that will help you to describe how you feel. We shall be using it throughout the interview to help you with questions about any area of your life. All you have to do is to point to the part of the chart that best describes how you feel, when you are asked. As you can see, it covers all of the feelings from when you are most satisfied with something or approve of it most strongly, to when you are least satisfied or most strongly disapprove.
>
> 'For example, if I asked you if you like hamburger, you might say "couldn't be better" if you really liked them a lot. This would show the strongest possible satisfaction or approval. On the other hand, if you hated hamburger, you might point to "couldn't be worse". This would show the strongest dissatisfaction. If you felt about equally satisfied and dissatisfied with hamburger, you would point to the middle of the chart, "mixed"; this would tell me that you were uncertain or of mixed feelings. As you can see, there is room for many shades of opinion in either direction.'

2.1   Enter an LSS score (between 1 and 7). When the patient is not capable of choosing one of the LSS categories, enter code 8 (not known).

Section 3: Work and education

3.1   Circle the client's answer. Here, as elsewhere, only one answer should be recorded per question; for example, '1', yes (the client 'agreed' with the statement); '2', no (the client 'disagreed' with the question); '3', DNK (the client 'did not know' or would not or could not answer). If the question is not applicable, score 8. This item includes paid employment, sheltered employment, all types of occupational therapies, and being a housewife/husband.

3.2   If the answer to 3.1 is 'yes', please list the occupation in the space provided.

3.3   Enter the number of hours.

3.4   Indicate the amount. If the patient does not know the gross salary, it is better to indicate an approximate amount rather than leaving the item blank. Try to use other sources of information (relatives, friends, patient's professional category, etc.) to obtain a figure. Only include the client's salary here: other sources of income such as state benefits are included in item 6.1.

3.5   Enter LSS score. This item assesses the client's principal activity, whether or not it is paid (for example, clients who are housewives or students).

3.6   Enter LSS score; if not applicable, enter code 8.

3.7   Enter LSS score. This item includes the possibilities not covered by item 3.5. Items 3.5 and 3.7 are mutually exclusive, so one of them necessarily has a score of 8.

Section 4: Leisure activities

4.1–5 Where a series of questions are asked, the scoring has been simplified to 1, yes; 2, no; 3, do not know/unwilling to answer. If not applicable, rate 8.

4.1   This includes going to a pub or bar to watch sport on television.

4.5   In this item 'were unable' covers both personal difficulties due to the illness and difficulties due to circumstances such as an excess of work.

4.6–8   Enter LSS score. Enter code 8 if not applicable or not known.

Section 5: Religion

5.1   Enter the code number for the appropriate listed religion. Agnostics are included in 'other' and atheists in 'none'.

5.2   Enter the number of services.

5.3   Enter LSS score. Satisfaction scored in this item relates to both religious faith and lack of it.

5.4   Enter LSS score. Satisfaction scored in this item is due to attending services or due to not attending services.

Section 6: Finances

6.1   Enter total income before deductions or payment of expenses. This item covers the total amount of the client's income, not just the salary from paid work (item 3.4). This includes benefits, help from family and so on. If the client does not want to reveal this information, try to use all possible sources to complete this item.

6.2   List the benefits. Try to use all possible sources of information to complete this item.

6.3   Circle the client's response. In this item and in 6.5 use the response categories 1, yes; 2, no; 3, do not know/unwilling to answer. If not applicable, rate 8.

6.4   Enter the amount required. This amount could vary according to whether the client lives alone or has to maintain a family.

6.5   Circle the client's response.

6.6–7   Enter LSS score.

Section 7: Living situation

7.1   Enter appropriate number from the options listed.

7.2   Enter number of months.

7.3   Enter number.

7.4   Circle client's response. In this item and in 7.5 use the response categories 1, yes; 2, no; 3, do not know/unwilling to answer. If not applicable, score 8.

7.5   Circle client's response.

7.6   Enter LSS score.

7.7   Enter LSS score. If the client lives alone, score for the satisfaction with the independence of living alone.

7.8   Enter LSS score. 'Influence' includes the influence that the client could exert both over fellow residents and over general life conditions, such as changing or organising the furniture, painting the walls, cleaning and meals.

7.9   Enter LSS score. Alternatively, rate the client's satisfaction with living alone.

7.10   Enter LSS score. Alternatively, rate the client's satisfaction with the privacy of living alone.

7.11   Enter LSS score.

7.12   Enter LSS score. If not applicable, score 8.

Section 8: Legal and safety

8.1–2 Circle the client's response. In these items use the response categories 1, yes; 2, no; 3, do not know/unwilling to answer. If not applicable, score 8.

8.2   Circle the client's response. It must be considered exclusively the client's subjective experience.

8.3–4 Enter LSS score.

Section 9: Family relations

9.1   Enter the code number for the options listed.

9.2   Enter the number.

9.3   Enter the code number for one of the options listed. Contact with relatives includes relatives who usually live with the client.

9.4   Circle client's response. Use the response categories 1, yes; 2, no; 3, do not know/unwilling to answer. If not applicable, score 8.

9.5   Enter LSS score.

9.6   Enter LSS score. 'Relatives' are defined as in 9.3.

9.7   Enter LSS score. If not applicable, score 8.

Section 10: Social relations

10.1   Circle client's response. In items 10.1–4 use the response categories 1, yes; 2, no; 3 do not know/unwilling to answer. If not applicable, score 8.

10.2–4 Circle client's response. Relatives are eligible to be considered as friends.

10.5   Enter LSS score.

10.6   Enter LSS score. If the client has no friend, score their satisfaction with this situation.

Section 11: Health

To rate the items in this section, all possible sources of information must be used (relatives, friends, medical records, etc.).

11.1   Circle client's response. In items 11.1–5 use the response categories 1, yes; 2, no; 3, do not know/unwilling to answer. If not applicable, score 8.

11.3   Circle client's response. If the client is currently an in-patient the score is 1 (yes).

11.4   Circle client's response.

11.5   Circle client's response.

11.6   Enter number of years.

11.7   Circle client's response, using the same response categories as items 11.1–5.

11.8–10   Enter LSS score.

11.11–20   Circle client's response, using the same response categories as items 11.1–5.

Section 12: Self-concept

Circle client's response for all items in this section, using the response categories 1, yes; 2, no; 3, do not know/unwilling to answer. If not applicable, score 8.

Section 13: General well-being

A suggested form of words for introducing this section is given in the questionnaire.

13.1   Enter LSS score.

13.2   Cantril's Ladder is a measure of global well-being scored by the client directly onto the questionnaire. Ask the client to look at the ladder and make a mark, preferably an X, at the point on the ladder that best expresses the client's level of life satisfaction; the mark need not rest on a rung, but must lie within the ladder, not next to it. The ladder is 100 mm long, regardless of the number of rungs; it is scored by measuring the distance in millimetres from the lowest rung of the ladder to the patient's mark. Enter the number of millimetres.

13.3   Enter the number of the listed item chosen.

13.4   List only one item per line.

Section 14: Final remarks

14.1   Circle the client's response, using the categories 1, yes; 2, no; 3, do not know/unwilling to answer. If not applicable, score 8.

Section 15: Interviewer comments

15.1   Enter the number of minutes.

15.2   Enter the number of the listed description chosen.

15.3   Complete the Quality of Life Uniscale by marking it with an 'X'.

Instructions for scoring

The LQoLP–EU can be conducted with severely ill mental patients in a variety of residential or community settings. The questionnaire should be administered by adequately trained professionals, and only those patients who have a florid psychopathological disorder, who are mute, or who have serious brain damage, could find themselves unable to complete it. The LQoLP–EU should be completed in a single interviewing session. Interviews are best conducted in a quiet place with sufficient privacy to allow the client to feel able to speak freely without being overheard. An environment free from interruptions is also highly desirable.

Subjective aspects are assessed using the seven-point Life Satisfaction Scale, rated by the client as described earlier in this chapter. The following scores can be obtained:

- Quality of life: average score of the nine domains comprising the items
  - work: 3.5–3.7
  - leisure: 4.6–4.8
  - religion: 5.3, 5.4
  - finance: 6.6, 6.7
  - living situation: 7.6–7.12
  - legal and safety: 8.4, 8.5
  - family relations: 9.5–9.7
  - social relations: 10.5, 10.6
  - health: 11.8–11.10.
- Perceived quality of life score: average of all the above dimensions.
- Psychological well-being
  - positive affect: 11.11–11.15, divided by the number of items (five)
  - negative affect: 11.16–11.20, divided by the number of items (five).
- Self-esteem
  - positive self-concept: 12.1, 12.2, 12.4, 12.6, 12.7 are summed and divided by the number of items (five)
  - negative self-concept: 12.3, 12.5, 12.8, 12.9, 12.10 are summed and divided by the number of items (five).
- Global well-being: average of items 2.1 and 13.1.
- Cantrill's Ladder: item 13.2.

Psychometric properties

One of the main objectives of the EPSILON Study (see Chapter 1) was the assessment of the psychometric properties of the different instruments in the five European languages. A detailed protocol describing the methods to be followed to verify their validity and reliability was elaborated (see Chapter 3).

After completing the LQoLP–EU it is possible to obtain a score reflecting the global quality of life of the person interviewed and scores for each of the domains composing the questionnaire. Only the items relating to the subjective perception of the client's own life are used for these scores.

Sub-scale for work

Average score of items 3.5, 3.6 and 3.7 (ratings 1–7). If item 3.1 was answered 'yes', average score of items 3.5 and 3.6 (sub-scale for employed), otherwise item 3.7 (sub-scale for unemployed).

Sub-scale for leisure

Average score of items 4.6, 4.7 and 4.8 (ratings 1–7).

Sub-scale for religion

Average score of items 5.3 and 5.4 (ratings 1–7).

Sub-scale for finance

Average score of items 6.6 and 6.7 (ratings 1–7).

Sub-scale for living situation

Average score of items 7.6–7.12 (ratings 1–7).

Sub-scale for legal and safety

Average score of items 8.3 and 8.4 (ratings 1–7).

Sub-scale for family relations

Average score of items 9.5, 9.6 and 9.7 (ratings 1–7).

Sub-scale for social relations

Average score of items 10.5 and 10.6 (ratings 1–7).

Sub-scale for health

Average score of items 11.8, 11.9 and 11.10 (ratings 1–7).

Perceived quality of life total

This measure is derived from summing the scores of the sub-scales for work, leisure, religion, finance, living situation, legal and safety, family relations, social relations and health, and dividing the total by the number of sub-scales (nine).

Sub-scale for general well-being

Average score of items 2.1 and 13.1 (ratings 1–7).

Ratings of affect

All items from 11.11 to 11.20 (inclusive) with missing data, not answered or answered with 'no' are recoded to 0. Four ratings are thus obtained:

- Rating of positive affect: scores for items 11.11–11.15 are summed and divided by the number of items (five).
- Rating of negative affect: scores for items 11.16–11.20 are summed and divided by the number of items (five).
- Affect balance for gross score:

  (11.11 + 11.12 + 11.13 + 11.14 + 11.15) – (11.16 + 11.17 + 11.18 + 11.19 + 11.20).
- Affect balance for average score: (positive affect score) – (negative affect score).

Self-concept score

All items from 12.1 to 12.10 (inclusive) with missing data, not answered or answered with 'no' are recoded to 0. Four ratings are thus obtained:

- Positive self-concept score: items 12.1, 12.2, 12.4, 12.6 and 12.7 are summed and divided by the number of items (five).
- Negative self-concept score: items 12.3, 12.5, 12.8, 12.9 and 12.10 are summed and divided by the number of items (five).
- Self-concept for gross score:

  (12.1 + 12.2 + 12.4 + 12.6 + 12.7) – (12.3 + 12.5 + 12.8 + 12.9 + 12.10).
- Self-concept for average score: (positive self-concept score) – (negative self-concept score).

14 Development and reliability of the LQoLP–EU

José Luis Vázquez-Barquero, Luis Gaite, Andrés Herrán, Dolors Serrano López, Deirdre Sierra-Biddle, Aart Schene, Mirella Ruggeri and Peter Huxley

The deinstitutionalisation that took place in the 1960s and 1970s in Western countries (Bachrach, 1970; Lamb, 1979) promoted interest in studying the quality of life of people with mental illness, and with it the need to develop and test valid and applicable instruments. A good example of this interest is the European Psychiatric Services: Inputs Linked to Outcome Domains and Needs (EPSILON) Study, in which one of the primary objectives was to develop and adapt, in five European countries, cross-cultural research instruments covering key areas of mental health assessment (see Chapter 1). This section describes the development and adaptation process of the European version of the Lancashire Quality of Life Profile (LQoLP–EU).

A fundamental step in the development of research tools is the establishment of an adequate definition of the concept to be covered, and also of the possible domains to be included in such a definition. This is particularly difficult to achieve in the area of quality of life, in which, as Liu (1976) has said, 'there are as many quality of life definitions as there are people'. Thus we see that Lehman (1983a) defined quality of life as 'the sense of well-being experienced by people under their current life conditions', whereas Oliver (1991) extended the concept to cover the 'total health and welfare' of the individual. Finally, the World Health Organization regards quality of life as an individual's perception of their position in life in the context of the culture and value systems in which they live and in relation to their goals, expectations, standard and concerns (World Health Organization, 1993). With this diversity of opinions, there are bound to be disagreements concerning the structure and contents of any instrument purporting to measure quality of life.

A second element in delineating the 'construct' of quality of life is the decision whether to establish a generic and universal concept, or one that is specific to a particular area of experience or disease. As a reflection of this dilemma, quality of life instruments tend to be classified as generic or disease-specific (Patrick & Deyo, 1989; Lehman & Burns, 1990). Generic scales are designed to be applied across various types of illness, as well as in different health interventions (McDowell & Newell, 1987; Patrick & Deyo, 1989). Widely used generic scales are the Sickness Impact Profile (Bergner *et al*, 1981) and the 36-item Short Form Health Survey (Ware, 1996). However, a possible disadvantage of these instruments is that they could underestimate – or completely miss – problems specific to particular diseases. To solve this deficiency, disease-specific scales have been developed such as the Quality of Life Interview (Lehman *et al*, 1982; Lehman, 1983a,b) and the Lancashire Quality of Life Profile (Oliver *et al*, 1996).

Finally, we should acknowledge that in mental health research, the assessment of quality of life should take into consideration both its subjective and objective components. Subjective quality of life reflects the patient's personal opinion and thus can only be measured by self-report. In this context, subjective quality of life, a central component of quality of life assessment, could be operationalised assessing life satisfaction as a whole and taking into consideration basic life domains such as personal circumstances, relationships and finances. Objective elements of quality of life are mainly based on economic or social indicators and therefore have little or no relation to subjective experience. Although the lack of correlation between objective measures and individuals' own perceptions justifies the inclusion of both elements in the assessment, the fact is that many researchers adopt in their studies the strategy of exclusively exploring the patient's living conditions and identifying objective indicators of quality of life, whereas others focus on exploring the subjective dimension (Awad *et al*, 1997).

These, among others, were the main issues taken into consideration in the process of developing the European version of the Lancashire Quality of Life Profile (LQoLP). The intention was to develop and test a psychosis-specific, cross-culturally applicable, easy-to-use and reliable assessment instrument, covering both objective and subjective dimensions of quality of life.

The original instrument

The original LQoLP was a structured self-report interview, comprising 105 items, designed to be administered by trained interviewers. It was developed by Oliver *et al* (1996) from Lehman's Quality of Life Interview (Lehman *et al*, 1982; Lehman, 1983a,b), combining objective and subjective measures in several life 'domains', four subject areas retained from Lehman's original interview, an additional life domain, and additional measures of global well-being, affect and self-esteem. The four areas retained were personal characteristics, objective quality of life indicators, subjective quality of life indicators and a global well-being measure. The objective and subjective indicators cover the eight original life domains – work and education (7 items), leisure and participation (8 items), finances (7 items), living situation (12 items), legal status and safety (5 items), family relations (7 items), social relations (6 items) and health (10 items) – with the addition of religion (4 items). These domains were derived originally by means of the critical incident technique, in which several thousand interviewees reported several thousand separate incidents that had had an impact on them, and which were then grouped into categories (Flanagan, 1982; Oliver *et al*, 1997). Objective well-being items are composed largely of social and economic indicators, and the subjective aspects of these domains are assessed using a modified version of the Lehman seven-point scale, which is rated by the respondent. This scale is identified in the interview as the Life Satisfaction Scale (LSS); a rating of 1 means life 'could not be worse', and 7 means life 'could not be better'.

In addition, the interview allows the assessment of the following areas: psychological well-being (10 items); self-esteem (10 items; Rosenberg, 1965); global well-being (3 items), including Cantril's ladder (Cantril, 1965), transformed from a 9-point categorical scale into a 100-point continuous scale; the Quality of Life Uniscale (Spitzer & Dobson, 1981), which evaluates the patient's quality of life independently of the patient's opinion; and the 'perceived quality of life' score, an average of the sum of the subjective items of the first nine domains. The LQoLP produces a profile made up of scores and separate global well-being assessments; it does not attempt to generate a single overall score to reflect the complexities of people's circumstances. The subjective well-being items follow on immediately after the objective questions in each life domain: this makes it clear to the respondent that a subjective response is sought, and avoids the 'halo' effect that might result if all the subjective well-being ratings were made in succession.

The psychometric properties of the LQoLP were assessed in people with chronic psychiatric illness. However, the reliability of the instrument was not verified, leaving a gap in the assessment of the psychometric properties of the instrument that needed to be filled. In addition, the LQoLP and its predecessor were developed from the perspective of English-speaking patients; verification of the cross-cultural applicability of the instrument in different European languages was therefore also required.

Development of the European version

The translation and adaptation process followed the procedure outlined in Chapter 2. The use of focus groups to assist in the cross-cultural adaptation allowed identification of conflictive areas in the items content, wording and cultural applicability of the instrument, leading to a number of changes in the translated versions (Knudsen *et al*, 2000). As a result of the experience obtained in the focus group and pilot testing of the instrument, a detailed manual was produced to clarify aspects related to its administration and scoring.

Validity

Construct, content and criterion validity of the LQoLP were assessed by Oliver *et al* (1996, 1997) and were considered good. In addition, the findings of the focus groups in the various EPSILON centres confirmed the high validity of the LQoLP–EU, with no substantial difference between centres.

Reliability

The reliability of the LQoLP–EU was specifically tested in the EPSILON Study, by verifying its internal consistency and test–retest reliability in different sites.

Internal consistency

The internal consistency was verified by computing Cronbach's α coefficient for each site separately, and inter-site differences were tested (Gaite *et al*, 2000). The α coefficients were high for Life Satisfaction Scale average scores (Table 14.1), with a pooled estimate of 0.87 (95% CI 0.85–0.88). The internal consistency of nine subjective life domains was in general adequate, but in four domains it was below 0.70: work (0.30), leisure activities (0.56), religion (0.62) and social relations (0.66). In the case of work, values differed between centres: the lowest were found in Amsterdam (0.12) and Santander (0.18) and the highest in London (0.76). The Pearson correlation between items in this domain was not significantly different from zero in either Amsterdam (0.107) or Santander (0.135). It has to be recognised that assessment of the internal consistency of this sub-domain is difficult, because of missing or inapplicable items. In the domain of religion, the most conflictive centre was Amsterdam, where α=0.33 (95% CI –0.15 to 0.58); this might be related to the fact that religion is a sensitive topic both for people with schizophrenia and for the general population. The Cronbach's α values for the affect balance and self-esteem scales were all satisfactory, although α was lower for negative self-esteem (0.67) than for positive self-esteem (0.77).

Test–retest reliability

Test–retest reliability was verified using intraclass correlation coefficients (ICCs). Table 14.2 shows the intraclass correlation between the test and retest interviews for the patients in the reliability sub-sample.

Table 14.1 Internal consistency of the Lancashire Quality of Life Profile – European Version: Cronbach's alpha coefficients

Sub-scales	Items	Pooled sample		Amsterdam		Copenhagen		London		Santander		Verona		Test of equality
		n	α (95% CI)	n	α (95% CI)	n	α (95% CI)	n	α (95% CI)	n	α (95% CI)	n	α (95% CI)	P
LSS score	24[1]	404	0.87 (0.85–0.88)	61	0.84 (0.77–0.89)	52	0.83 (0.75–0.89)	84	0.86 (0.81–0.89)	100	0.83 (0.77–0.87)	107	0.90 (0.87–0.92)	0.11
Work	2	404	0.30 (0.14–0.42)	61	0.12 (−0.50–0.45)	52	0.64 (0.35–0.78)	84	0.76 (0.62–0.84)	100	0.18 (−0.23–0.44)	107	0.47 (0.20–0.63)	<0.01
Leisure activities	3	404	0.56 (0.48–0.62)	61	0.67 (0.47–0.78)	52	0.29 (0.15–0.55)	84	0.66 (0.51–0.76)	100	0.42 (0.17–0.58)	107	0.62 (0.47–0.72)	0.07
Religion	2	404	0.62 (0.53–0.68)	61	0.33 (−0.15–0.58)	52	0.48 (0.05–0.69)	84	0.92 (0.87–0.94)	100	0.71 (0.56–0.80)	107	0.62 (0.42–0.74)	<0.01
Finances	2	404	0.88 (0.85–0.90)	61	0.72 (0.53–0.83)	52	0.93 (0.87–0.95)	84	0.98 (0.96–0.98)	100	0.88 (0.82–0.91)	107	0.85 (0.78–0.89)	<0.01
Living situation	6	404	0.85 (0.82–0.87)	61	0.78 (0.68–0.85)	52	0.75 (0.62–0.84)	84	0.94 (0.91–0.95)	100	0.74 (0.65–0.81)	107	0.86 (0.81–0.89)	<0.01
Safety	2	404	0.82 (0.78–0.85)	61	0.79 (0.64–0.87)	52	0.79 (0.63–0.87)	84	0.96 (0.93–0.97)	100	0.68 (0.52–0.78)	107	0.81 (0.72–0.87)	<0.01
Family relations	2	404	0.80 (0.75–0.83)	61	0.69 (0.46–0.80)	52	0.72 (0.49–0.83)	84	0.91 (0.86–0.94)	100	0.92 (0.88–0.94)	107	0.65 (0.48–0.76)	<0.01
Social relations	2	404	0.66 (0.58–0.72)	61	0.65 (0.39–0.78)	52	0.58 (0.25–0.75)	84	0.56 (0.30–0.70)	100	0.49 (0.22–0.65)	107	0.83 (0.75–0.88)	0.02
Health	3	404	0.74 (0.69–0.78)	61	0.72 (0.57–0.82)	52	0.66 (0.44–0.78)	84	0.79 (0.69–0.85)	100	0.66 (0.52–0.76)	107	0.75 (0.65–0.82)	0.49
Global well-being	2	398	0.83 (0.79–0.86)	61	0.75 (0.56–0.85)	50	0.83 (0.69–0.90)	83	0.94 (0.91–0.96)	100	0.82 (0.72–0.87)	106	0.79 (0.69–0.86)	<0.01
Positive affect	5	402	0.74 (0.70–0.78)	61	0.71 (0.56–0.81)	51	0.71 (0.55–0.81)	84	0.64 (0.49–0.74)	100	0.70 (0.59–0.78)	106	0.83 (0.77–0.88)	<0.01
Negative affect	5	401	0.68 (0.62–0.72)	61	0.58 (0.36–0.72)	50	0.66 (0.46–0.78)	84	0.72 (0.60–0.80)	100	0.66 (0.54–0.75)	106	0.68 (0.56–0.76)	<0.01
Positive self-esteem	5	403	0.77 (0.73–0.80)	61	0.71 (0.56–0.80)	51	0.78 (0.66–0.86)	84	0.81 (0.73–0.86)	100	0.70 (0.59–0.78)	107	0.81 (0.74–0.86)	0.35
Negative self-esteem	5	402	0.67 (0.62–0.72)	61	0.64 (0.46–0.76)	50	0.74 (0.59–0.83)	84	0.45 (0.23–0.61)	100	0.75 (0.66–0.82)	107	0.74 (0.65–0.81)	0.04

LSS, Life Satisfaction Scale.
1. Three items were excluded from this analysis since they are utilised exclusively in specific situations ('if applicable'): for people married, retired or with previous hospitalisations.

Table 14.2 Test–retest reliability of the Lancashire Quality of Life Profile – European Version (LQoLP–EU) summary scores in the pooled sample and by site

Sub-scale	Items	Pooled $n=264$		Amsterdam $n=51$		Copenhagen $n=46$		London $n=51$		Santander $n=50$		Verona $n=66$		Test of equality of ICCs (P)
		ICC	(s.e.)$_m$	ICC	(s.e.)$_m$	ICC	(s.e.)$_m$	ICC	(s.e.)$_m$	ICC	(s.e.)$_m$	ICC	(s.e.)$_m$	
LSS score	27	0.82	0.29	0.86	0.24	0.83	0.28	0.82	0.24	0.85	0.24	0.77	0.41	0.65
Work situation	3	0.66	0.76	0.73	0.63	0.38	0.92	0.65	0.62	0.82	0.61	0.61	0.94	0.01
Leisure activities	3	0.68	0.56	0.79	0.51	0.62	0.54	0.61	0.53	0.68	0.55	0.67	0.67	0.34
Religion	2	0.62	0.67	0.51	0.88	0.71	0.64	0.58	0.66	0.74	0.51	0.54	0.69	0.24
Finances	2	0.72	0.73	0.72	0.69	0.73	0.74	0.87	0.42	0.81	0.69	0.56	1.04	<0.01
Living situation	7	0.75	0.51	0.67	0.51	0.67	0.55	0.87	0.42	0.79	0.39	0.65	0.63	<0.01
Safety	2	0.61	0.74	0.64	0.75	0.76	0.51	0.72	0.63	0.71	0.62	0.32	1.06	<0.01
Family relations	3	0.66	0.73	0.15	0.64	0.71	0.75	0.73	0.64	0.59	0.86	0.61	0.86	0.15
Social relations	2	0.65	0.67	0.75	0.61	0.72	0.66	0.52	0.57	0.81	0.48	0.51	0.93	<0.01
Health	3	0.71	0.56	0.81	0.42	0.71	0.59	0.65	0.54	0.75	0.49	0.65	0.68	0.27
Global well-being	2	0.78	0.58	0.73	0.64	0.83	0.45	0.72	0.59	0.81	0.56	0.81	0.62	0.36
Positive affect	5	0.72	0.16	0.82	0.14	0.61	0.19	0.79	0.13	0.81	0.12	0.61	0.21	0.05
Negative affect	5	0.71	0.16	0.66	0.15	0.79	0.13	0.61	0.20	0.81	0.14	0.75	0.17	0.07
Positive self-esteem	5	0.71	0.16	0.68	0.14	0.83	0.13	0.73	0.17	0.41	0.19	0.77	0.14	<0.01
Negative self-esteem	5	0.63	0.18	0.57	0.21	0.73	0.15	0.49	0.19	0.72	0.18	0.66	0.18	0.10
Cantril's Ladder	1	0.65	13.49	0.59	15.09	0.85	9.36	0.81	9.64	0.64	15.03	0.38	17.54	<0.01
QoL Uniscale	1	0.81	7.61	0.72	7.81	0.75	9.05	0.85	6.85	0.91	5.83	0.49	13.92	<0.05

ICC, intraclass correlation coefficient; (s.e.)$_m$, standard error of measurement (square root of error component of variance); LSS; Life Satisfaction Scale; QoL, Quality of Life.

For this evaluation, data from only 294 patients were used. The pooled ICC score for global satisfaction (LSS) was 0.82. The nine life domain sub-scale ICC values ranged from 0.61 (safety) to 0.75 (living situation). The ICC estimates for the affect balance scale were 0.72 for positive affect and 0.71 for negative affect. In the self-esteem scale the results were 0.71 for positive self-esteem and 0.63 for negative self-esteem. Test–retest reliabilities were 0.65 for Cantril's Ladder, 0.78 for global well-being and 0.81 for QoL Uniscale.

Test–retest ICCs were good for the LSS (pooled estimate 0.82, 95% CI 0.78–0.85) and also for the individual sub-scales, which ranged from 0.61 to 0.75. The coefficients appear to be higher for the LSS than for the individual sub-scales, perhaps because of the greater stability of the LSS, being the total of many items. There is evidence for differences between sites for the individual sub-scales, but not for the LSS. The only centre with relatively low ICCs for sub-scales is Verona, but paired *t*-tests on the time 2 and time 1 results show this is not due to an overall tendency to higher or lower values at retest in Verona, but can be explained by random variation. There are relatively high values of the standard error of measurement (s.e.)$_m$ associated with the low ICCs at Verona, and the higher (s.e.)$_m$ in Verona is the explanation for the overall higher standard deviation (0.84). This also seems to be the case for the low ICC for the religion sub-scale in Amsterdam. The test–retest ICC for the total subjective satisfaction score was good, and ICCs were adequate for each of the nine life domains. Although there was some evidence of differences between the sites in the reliabilities of the sub-domains, they were all above 0.61. The total score showed no evidence of differences, and a pooled estimate was 0.82 (95% CI 0.79–0.86). Finally, paired *t*-tests analysis between interviews at time 1 and time 2 showed that there was no overall tendency to higher or lower values at retest, indicating that the values between test and retest are reasonably stable. Therefore it seems that the time between the test and the retest is not long enough to influence the results; furthermore, there seems to be no tendency for patients to modify their appraisal of quality of life in the second interview (i.e. because answering the questions makes them reassess their quality of life).

Conclusions

The Lancashire Quality of Life Profile – European Version has proved to be a satisfactory instrument for measuring quality of life in different European settings. It has good internal consistency and reliability. Furthermore, it is 'user-friendly', takes about half an hour to administer (on average) and is available in Danish, Dutch, English, Italian and Spanish, each accompanied by a manual clarifying the use of the instrument in the different settings.

References and further reading

Awad, A. G., Voruganti, L. N. & Heslegrave, R. J. (1997) Measuring quality of life in patients with schizophrenia. *Pharmacoeconomics*, **11**, 32–47.

Bachrach, L. L. (ed.) (1970) *Deinstitutionalization: An Analytic Review and Sociological Perspective*. Rockville, MD: National Institute of Mental Health.

Bergner, M., Bobbitt, R. A., Carter, W. B., et al (1981) The Sickness Impact Profile: development and final revision of a health status measure. *Medical Care*, **19**, 787–805.

Cantril, H. (ed.) (1965) *The Pattern of Human Concerns*. New Brunswick, NJ: Rutgers University Press.

Flanagan, J. C. (1982) Measurement of quality of life: current state of the art. *Archives of Physical Medicine and Rehabilitation*, **63**, 56–59.

Gaite, L., Vázquez-Barquero, J. L., Arrizabalaga, A. A., et al (2000) Quality of life in schizophrenia: development, reliability and internal consistency of the Lancashire Quality of Life Profile – European Version. EPSILON Study 8. *British Journal of Psychiatry*, **177** (suppl. 39), s49–s54.

Knudsen, H. C., Vázquez-Barquero, J. L., Welcher, B., et al (2000) Translation and cross-cultural adaptation of outcome measurements for schizophrenia. EPSILON Study 2. *British Journal of Psychiatry*, **177** (suppl. 39), s8–s14.

Lamb, R. H. (1979) The new asylums in the community. *Archives of General Psychiatry*, **36**, 129–134.

Lehman, A. F. (1983a) The well-being of chronic mental patients: assessing their quality of life. *Archives of General Psychiatry*, **40**, 369–373.

Lehman, A. F. (1983b) The effects of psychiatric symptoms on quality of life assessments among the chronic mentally ill. *Evaluation and Program Planning*, **6**, 143–151.

Lehman, A. F. & Burns, B. J. (1990) Severe mental illness in the community. In *Quality of Life Assessments in Clinical Trials* (ed. B. Spilker), pp. 357–366. New York: Raven Press.

Lehman, A., Ward, N. & Linn, L. (1982) Chronic mental patients: the quality of life issue. *American Journal of Psychiatry*, **139**, 1271–1276.

Liu, B. (1976) *Quality of Life Indicators in U.S. Metropolitan Areas: A Statistical Analysis*. New York: Praeger.

McDowell, I. & Newell, C. (1987) *Measuring Health: A Guide to Rating Scales and Questionnaires*. New York: Oxford University Press.

Norusis, M. (1993) *SPSS for Windows*. Chicago: SPSS Inc.

Oliver, J. (1991) The social care directive: development of a quality of life profile for use in community services for the mentally ill. *Social Work and Social Sciences Review*, **3**, 5–45.

Oliver, J., Huxley, P., Bridges, K., et al (1996) *Quality of Life and Mental Health Services*. London: Routledge.

Oliver, J., Huxley, P., Priebe, S., et al. (1997) Measuring the quality of life of severely ill people using the Lancashire Quality of Life Profile. *Social Psychiatry and Psychiatric Epidemiology*, **32**, 76–83.

Patrick, D. L. & Deyo, R. A. (1989) Generic and disease-specific measures in assessing health status and quality of life. *Medical Care*, **17** (suppl.) s217–s232.

Rosenberg, M. (ed.) (1965) *Society and the Adolescent Self-image*. Princeton: Princeton University Press.

Spitzer, W. O. & Dobson, A. J. (1981) Measuring the quality of life of cancer patients. *Journal of Chronic Disorders*, **34**, 585–597.

Ware, J. E. J. (1996) The SF-36 health survey. In *Quality of Life and Pharmacoeconomics in Clinical Trials* (ed. B. Spilker), pp. 337–345. Philadelphia: Lippincott/Raven.

World Health Organization (1993) *WHOQOL: Study Protocol*. Geneva: WHO.

15 Lancashire Quality of Life Profile – European Version

Luis Gaite, José Luis Vázquez-Barquero, Jo Oliver
and Peter Huxley

Lancashire Quality of Life Profile – European Version

Centre/Country _____ Client study number ☐☐☐ Date (dd/mm/yy) ☐☐/☐☐/☐☐

Interviewer's code ☐

If the client declines to be interviewed, please state the reason(s) and stop here:

Starting time: _____

1 Client's personal details

1.1	Age	Years	☐☐
1.2	Gender	1 Male	☐
		2 Female	

1.3 Ethnic group
- a White
- b Black Caribbean
- c Black African
- d Black other
- e Indian
- f Pakistani
- g Bangladeshi
- h Chinese
- i Other ☐

1.4 Age on leaving full-time education   Years ☐

2 General well-being

2.1 Can you describe how you feel about your life as a whole today? (LSS: 1–7) ☐

3 Work/education

3.1 Do you have a job?
- 1 Yes
- 2 No
- 3 Don't know ☐

3.2 If yes, what is your occupation? _____

3.3 How many hours per week do you work?   Hours ☐☐

3.4 How much money are you paid weekly (gross)? _____

How satisfied are you with: **(Life Satisfaction Scale 1–7)**

3.5 your job (or sheltered employment; occupational or industrial therapy; studies) ☐

3.6 the amount of money that you make ☐

3.7 being unemployed or retired (if appropriate) ☐

4   Participation in leisure activities

In the past fortnight, have you: (1=Yes   2=No   3=Don't know)

4.1   been out to play or watch a sport?

4.2   been out shopping?

4.3   been for a ride in a bus, car or train other than to go to and from work?

4.4   watched television or listened to the radio?

4.5   In the past **year**, have there been times when you would have liked to have had more leisure activity but were unable?

How satisfied are you with: **(Life Satisfaction Scale 1–7)**

4.6   the amount of pleasure you get from things you do at home?

4.7   the amount of pleasure you get from things you do outside your home?

4.8   the pleasure you get from radio or TV?

5.   Religion

5.1   What is your religion now?

1 Protestant
2 Roman Catholic
3 Jewish
4 Muslim
5 Hindu
6 Other
7 None

5.2   How often have you attended religious services in the past month?

Number of times

How satisfied are you with: **(Life Satisfaction Scale 1–7)**

5.3   your religious faith and its teachings (or with the absence of them)

5.4   the frequency that you attend services (includes no attending)

6.   Finances

6.1   What is your total weekly income?

6.2   Which, if any, state benefits do you receive?

6.3   In the past year, have you been turned down for any state benefits for which you have applied? **(1=Yes   2=No   3=Don't know)**

6.4   About how much money per week do you need to be able to live as you would wish?

6.5   During the past year, have you ever lacked
       the money to enjoy everyday life?   **(1 = Yes   2 = No   3 = Don't know)**

How satisfied are you with: **(Life Satisfaction Scale 1–7)**

6.6   how well-off you are financially?

6.7   the amount of money you have to spend on enjoyment?

7.   Living situation

7.1   What is your current residence?

1 Hostel
2 Boarding out
3 Group home
4 Hospital ward
5 Sheltered housing
6 Private house (owner-occupied)
7 Private house (rented)
8 Flat
9 Other
10 None

7.2   How long have you lived there?   Months

7.3   How many other people live here?   Number of people

7.4   Do your family live here too?   **(1 = Yes   2 = No   3 = Don't know)**

7.5   In the past year, have there been times when
       you wanted to move or improve your living
       conditions but were unable to do so?   **(1 = Yes   2 = No   3 = Don't know)**

How satisfied were you with: **Life Satisfaction Scale 1–7**

7.6   the living arrangements here?

7.7   the amount of independence you have here?

7.8   the amount of influence you have here?

7.9   living with the people who you do?

7.10   the amount of privacy that you have here?

7.11   the prospect of living here for a long time?

7.12   the prospect of returning to live in a hospital? (if applicable)

8.   Legal and safety

In the past year, have you been: **(1 = Yes   2 = No   3 = Don't know)**

8.1(a) accused of a crime?

8.1(b) assaulted, beaten, molested or otherwise a
        victim of violence?
        (rate only if there has been physical contact)

| 8.2 | In the past year, have there been any times when you would have liked police or legal help but were unable to get it? | (1=Yes   2=No   3=Don't know) | ☐ |

How satisfied are you with: (Life Satisfaction Scale 1–7)

| 8.3 | your general personal safety? | ☐ |
| 8.4 | the safety of this neighbourhood? | ☐ |

9.   Family relations

| 9.1 | What is your current marital status? | 1 Married/living with a partner
2 Single
3 Widowed
4 Divorced
5 Separated
6 Other | ☐ |

| 9.2 | How many children do you have? | Number of children: | ☐☐ |

| 9.3 | How often do you have contact with a relative? | 1 Daily
2 Weekly
3 Monthly
4 Annually
5 Less than annually
6 Not appropriate/don't know | ☐ |

| 9.4 | In the past year, have there been times when you would have liked to have participated in family activities but were unable? | (1=Yes   2=No   3=Don't know) | ☐ |

How satisfied are you with: (Life Satisfaction Scale 1–7)

9.5	your family in general?	☐
9.6	the amount of contact you have with your relatives?	☐
9.7	your marriage? (if applicable)	☐

10.   Social relations

People differ in how much friendship they need   (1=Yes   2=No   3=Don't know)

10.1	Would you say that you are the sort of person who can manage without friends?	☐
10.2	Do you have anyone who you would call a 'close friend' (who knows you very well)?	☐
10.3	Do you have a friend to whom you could turn for help if you needed it?	☐
10.4	In the past week, have you visited a friend?	☐

How satisfied are you with: **(Life Satisfaction Scale 1–7)**

10.5   the way that you get on with other people?

10.6   the number of friends you have?

11.   Health

During the past year, have you: **(1=Yes   2=No   3=Don't know)**

11.1   seen a doctor for a physical illness?

11.2   seen a doctor for your nerves?

11.3   been in hospital for your nerves?

11.4   taken medication for your nerves?

11.5   Do you have a physical disability that affects your mobility?

11.6   How old were you when you were first
        admitted to a psychiatric hospital/ward
        (if appropriate)   Age in years:

11.7   In the past **year**, have there been times when
        you wanted help from a doctor or other
        professional for your health but were unable
        to get it?   **(1=Yes   2=No   3=Don't know)**

How satisfied are you with   **(Life Satisfaction Scale 1–7)**

11.8   your general state of health?

11.9   how often you see a doctor?

11.10   your nervous well-being?

During the past month, did you ever feel: **(1=Yes   2=No   3=Don't know)**

11.11   pleased about having accomplished something?

11.12   that things were going your way?

11.13   proud because someone complimented you on something you have done?

11.14   particularly excited or interested in something?

11.15   'on top of the world'?

11.16   too restless to sit in a chair?

11.17   bored?

11.18   depressed or very unhappy?

11.19   very lonely or remote from other people?

11.20   upset because someone criticised you?

12. Self-concept

How satisfied we are with ourselves is also a very important part of our lives. Do you agree that the following statements apply to you?

12.1   You feel that you are a person of worth, at least on an equal plane with others

12.2   You feel that you have a number of good qualities

12.3   All in all, you are inclined to feel that you are a failure

12.4   You are able to do things as well as most others

12.5   You feel you do not have much to be proud of

12.6   You take a positive attitude towards yourself

12.7   On the whole, you are satisfied with yourself

12.8   You wish you could have more respect for yourself

12.9   You certainly feel useless at times

12.10 At times you think you are no good at all

13. General well-being

During the course of this interview, we have discussed many of the conditions of your life and how you feel about them. Might we try and sum them up now?

13.1   Can you tell me how you feel about your life as a whole?   **(Life Satisfaction Scale 1–7)**

13.2   This is a picture of a ladder. I would like you to imagine that the bottom of the ladder represents the very worst outcome that you could expect to have had in life. The top represents the very best outcome you could have expected.

Please mark with a ✗ where on this ladder you would put your life at present.
(Ask client to mark ladder)

Best possible outcome

Worst possible outcome

13.3 How happy has your life been overall?

1 Very happy
2 Pretty happy
3 Average
4 Not happy
5 Don't know

13.4 Can you name any thing(s) that would improve the quality of your life?

1. _____
   _____

2. _____
   _____

3. _____
   _____

14. Final remarks

Thank you for having spoken to me in such an honest and open way about your life.

14.1 We may wish to contact you again in future, perhaps next year. Would you be willing to be interviewed again? **(1=Yes   2=No   3=Don't know)**

Thank you very much for your cooperation.

Finishing time: _____

15. Interviewer comments

Before filing this questionnaire or proceeding to the next interview, please complete the following section while your impressions of both the client and the setting for the interview are still fresh in your memory.

15.1 How long did the interview take? Time in minutes: _____

15.2 How reliable or unreliable do you think the client's responses were?

1 Very reliable

2 Generally reliable

3 Generally unreliable

4 Very unreliable

15.3 Please complete the QUALITY OF LIFE UNISCALE now. Mark with a ✗ the appropriate place within the box to indicate your rating of this person's present quality of life.

Lowest quality applies to someone completely dependent physically on others, seriously mentally disabled, unaware of surroundings and in a hopeless position.

Highest quality applies to someone physically and mentally independent, communicating well with others, able to do most things, enjoying pulling their weight, with a hopeful yet realistic attitude.

Lowest quality [   ] Highest quality

Thank you for your help

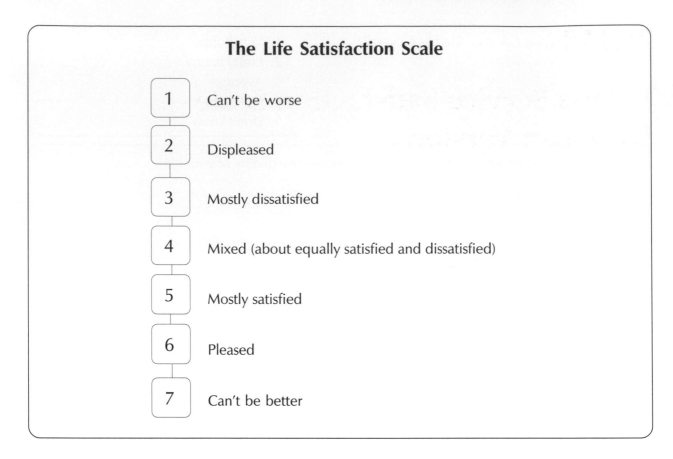

The Life Satisfaction Scale

1   Can't be worse

2   Displeased

3   Mostly dissatisfied

4   Mixed (about equally satisfied and dissatisfied)

5   Mostly satisfied

6   Pleased

7   Can't be better

Part VI

Verona Service Satisfaction Scale – European Version

16 Introduction and manual for the VSSS–EU

Antonio Lasalvia, Rosa Bruna Dall'Agnola, Doriana Cristofalo, Thomas Greenfield and Mirella Ruggeri

The Verona Service Satisfaction Scale (VSSS) is a setting-specific, validated, multidimensional scale for measuring patients' satisfaction with mental health services. It was first developed in an 82-item version (Ruggeri & Dall'Agnola, 1993), consisting of a set of 37 items cross-setting for health services, and a set of 45 items specific for mental health services: the former group of items involved aspects meant *a priori* to be relevant across a broad array of both medical and psychiatric settings, and was derived from the *Service Satisfaction Scale (SSS–30)* developed by a team at the University of California, San Francisco (Greenfield & Attkisson, 1989, 2004; Attkisson & Greenfield, 1994; Ruggeri & Greenfield, 1995); the latter group of items involved aspects relevant specifically in mental health settings, particularly in community-based services, such as social skills and types of intervention (e.g. admissions, psychotherapy, rehabilitation) and has been developed on purpose by the authors of the VSSS, also informed in part by family and community-residential versions of the SSS–30 (Ruggeri & Greenfield, 1995).

The original VSSS–82, in its versions for parents and relatives, has been tested for acceptability, content validity, sensitivity and test–retest reliability, showing good psychometric properties (Ruggeri *et al*, 1994). Factor analysis was also performed (Ruggeri *et al*, 1996), and a combination of results obtained in the validation study and factor analysis has given origin to the *intermediate* (VSSS–54) and the *short* version (VSSS–32, two reliable instruments that can be easily used in everyday clinical settings.

The European version (EU version) of the questionnaire was developed from the VSSS–54, between 1997 and 2000, in the context of the EPSILON Study (Becker *et al*, 1999). The EPSILON Study, the acronym for which was derived from *European Psychiatric Services: Inputs Linked to Outcome Domain and Needs*, was an EU Biomed–2 founded research project, intended to produce standardised versions of a series of key instruments, one of which was the VSSS–EU, in five languages (Spanish, Italian, English, German, Danish). Details on the instrument development process, which included translation, cross-cultural adaptation and reliability testing, are given in Ruggeri *et al* (2000). As a part of the process, and in order to maximise the reliability and validity of the instrument in a variety of cross-cultural settings, the present *Manual of Use* was developed. This manual was further refined, taking into consideration the experience acquired in the issue of the instrument, after the compilation of the EPSILON Study. Like its predecessor instruments, much of the format and item content of the VSSS–EU derives from the SSS–30 developed earlier (Greenfield & Attkisson, 1989), as well as versions of the SSS used in community- and hospital-based mental health programmes; see also Greenfield & Attkisson (2000, 2004) and Attkisson & Greenfield (1996), where the SSS–30 instrument is provided as an appendix.

The VSSS–EU is a reliable instrument for use in comparative cross-national research projects, as well as in routine clinical practice in mental health services across Europe. Results on satisfaction with mental health services among people with schizophrenia in five European countries are reported in Ruggeri *et al* (2003). The VSSS–EU has been specifically designed for community-based mental health services run by multidisciplinary teams of psychiatrists, psychologists, social workers and nurses. These services are assumed to have various treatment options (e.g. hospitalisation, day-care, rehabilitation, psychotherapy, home help, out-patient visits) available within the service or provided by various services that closely cooperate. The VSSS–EU may be easily adapted to community settings that differ slightly from this model (e.g. fewer treatment options or different composition of the care personnel), but caution should be used if the service organisation is radically different from the model assumed.

Conceptually, the items in VSSS–EU cover seven dimensions, which are made up of a certain number of items exploring various aspects of satisfaction with services:

- The *Overall Satisfaction* dimension is constituted by 3 items (11, 20, 21), which cover general aspects of satisfaction with mental health services
- The *Professionals' Skills and Behaviour* dimension is constituted by 24 items (2, 3a, 3b, 5a, 5b, 6a, 6b, 7, 10, 16a, 16b, 17, 18, 22a, 22b, 25a, 25b, 28, 33, 35a, 35b, 37a, 37b, 40), which cover various aspects of satisfaction with the professionals' behaviour such as technical skills, interpersonal skills, cooperation between service providers, respect of patients' rights, etc. Psychiatrists, psychologists, nurses and social workers are assessed in separate items.
- The *Information* dimension consists of 3 items (12, 19, 29), which cover aspects related to satisfaction with information on services, disorders and therapies.
- The *Access* dimension consists of 2 items (4, 8), which cover aspects related to satisfaction with service location, physical layout and costs.
- The *Efficacy* dimension consists of 8 items (1, 9, 13, 24, 26, 31, 34, 38), which cover aspects related to satisfaction with overall efficacy of the service, and service efficacy on specific aspects such as symptoms, social skills and family relationships.
- The *Types of Intervention* dimension consists of 17 items (14, 15, 39, 41–54), which cover various aspects of satisfaction with mental health care, such as drugs prescription, response to emergency, psychotherapy, rehabilitation, domicilliary care, admissions, housing, recreational activities, work, benefits, etc.
- The *Relative's Involvement* dimension consists of 6 items (23, 27, 30a, 30b, 32, 36), which cover various aspects of the patient's satisfaction with help given to his/her closest relative, such as listening, understanding, advice, information, help coping with the patient's problems, etc.

Instructions for item scoring

The VSSS–EU is designed for self-administration and can be completed without prior training. In cases of cognitive deficit, severe psychopathology or low level of literacy, a research worker may assist the patient and/or the relative by reading through the items with them. Special care must be taken to guarantee confidentiality and anonymity and, in the case of assisted administration, to stress the independence of the research worker from the clinical team. Questionnaire administration takes 20–30 minutes.

In the VSSS–EU, subjects are asked to express their overall feeling about their experience of the mental health service they have been attending in the past year.

Items 1–40 are rated on the following 5-point Likert scale:

1 = terrible
2 = mostly dissatisfied

> 3 = mixed
> 4 = mostly satisfied
> 5 = excellent

In the various items, the scoring is presented with alternate directionality to reduce stereotypic response.

Items 1–40 are based upon the assumption that the patient has a close caring relative often in contact with the service or that the patient is cared for by a multidisciplinary team, with separate assessment for psychiatrists'/psychologists' and social workers'/nurses' performance. If some of these items are not applicable, the research worker assisting the VSSS–EU administration should write 'N.A.' beside those specific items.

Items 41–54 consist of three questions:

> *Question A:* 'Did you receive the intervention x in the past year?' (yes/no/don't know).

If the answer is 'yes', the subject is asked:

> *Question B:* his/her rating of intervention on a 5-point Likert scale (1=terrible; 5=excellent).

If the answer is 'no', he/she is asked:

> *Question C:* 'do you think you would have liked to receive intervention x?' (6=no, 7=don't know, 8=yes).

For items 41–54, the research worker assisting the VSSS–EU administration should identify the kinds of intervention that are not provided by that specific mental health service and consider the corresponding items non-applicable. Therefore, before starting the data collection, the research worker should delete these non-applicable items (e.g. by crossing them out with a pen), in order to avoid patient misunderstandings. Researchers should be cautious in deleting items (also for the interventions that are not provided by the service assessed), because the VSSS–EU from this point of view can provide interesting information about the underprovision of care (e.g. about the patient's wish to receive an intervention that actually is not available).

For items 41–54, answers to the three questions can either be treated separately or collapsed into a single rating.

(a)   Where answers are treated separately:

Answers to *Question A* give a profile of the type of interventions provided. The following re-coding strategy may be useful:

> Ratings from 6–8 = 0 (intervention not provided);
> Ratings from 1–5 = 1 (intervention provided).

Answers to *Question B* (ratings 1–5) assess satisfaction with interventions provided.

Answers to Question C (ratings 6–8) assess satisfaction with the professionals' choice not to provide that intervention and give information on underprovision of care according to the patient's views. In this case, rating 6 will give the profile of interventions not provided but also not wanted. Rating 8 will instead give the profile of interventions not provided but wanted.

(b)   in order to collapse ratings obtained in questions A, B and C into a single rating, the following re-codings should be made:

> rating 6=4
> rating 8=2
> rating 7=missing

This rating will represent overall satisfaction with the management of this intervention, whether the intervention has been provided or not.

Data analysis

1. VSSS–EU mean total score

The VSSS–EU mean total score is obtained by summing up all items' values (if all items are applicable) and dividing by 63.

   If some items are not applicable, a global score is obtained by summing up all the items' values and dividing by the number of items assessed.

2. VSSS–EU mean dimension scores

Scores for each dimension are obtained by summing up all item values and then dividing by the number of items in each dimension as follows:

Overall satisfaction (3 items)
(items 11+20+21)/3

Professionals' skills and behaviour (24 items)
(items 2+3a+3b+5a+5b+6a+6b+7+10+16a+16b+17+18+22a+22b+25a+25b+28+33+35a +35b+37a+ 37b+40)/24

Information (3 items)
(items 12+19+29)/3

Access (2 items)
(items 4+8)/2

Efficacy (8 items)
(items 1+9+13+24+26+31+34+38)/8

Types of intervention (17 items)
(items 14+15+39+41+42+43+44+45+46+47+48+49+50+51+52+53+54)/17

Relative's involvement (6 items)
(items 23+27+30a+30b+32+36)/6

As for the VSSS–EU total mean score, if some items are not applicable, each dimension score is obtained by summing up all the items' values and dividing by the number of the items assessed. This approach, resulting in mean item-mean scores, prorated for the non-missing items, allows between-scale comparisons using the metric of the original response options, aiding interpretation.

   Frequency distributions may be analysed for the original ratings or for collapsed ratings. If they are collapsed, ratings may be re-coded on the basis of a strict or a broad criterion of dissatisfaction, depending on the research purpose.

Strict criterion

ratings 1 and 2 = 1 (dissatisfied)
rating 3 = 2 (mixed)
rating 4 and 5 = 3 (satisfied)

Broad criterion

ratings 1, 2 and 3 = 1 (dissatisfied)
ratings 4 and 5 = 2 (satisfied)

Use of the broad criterion may help to minimise bias due to users' difficulty in expressing dissatisfaction overtly.

References and further reading

Attkisson, C. C. & Greenfield, T. K. (1994) The Client Satisfaction Questionnaire–8 and the Services Satisfaction Questionnaire–30. In *Psychological Testing: Treatment Planning and Outcome Assessment* (ed. M. Maruish), pp. 404–420. San Francisco: Lawrence Erlbaum Associates.

Attkisson, C. C. & Greenfield, T. K. (1996) The Client Satisfaction Questionnaire (CSQ) scales and the Service Satisfaction Scale–30 (SSS–30). In *Outcomes Assessment in Clinical Practice* (eds L. I. Sederer & B. Dickey), pp. 120–127. Baltimore, MD: Williams & Wilkins.

Attkisson, C. C., Greenfield, T. K. & Melendez, D. (1995) *The Client Satisfaction Questionnaire (CSQ) Scales and Service Satisfaction Scales (SSS): A History of Scale Development and a Guide for Users*. San Francisco, CA: Department of Psychiatry, University of California. http://saawww.ucsf.edu/csq/CSQMANU.htm

Becker, T., Knapp, M., Knudsen, H. C., *et al* and the EPSILON Study Group (1999) The EPSILON study of schizophrenia in five European countries: design and methodology for standardising outcome measures and comparing patterns of care and service costs. *British Journal of Psychiatry*, **175**, 514–521.

Greenfield, T. K. & Attkisson, C. C. (1989) Steps toward a multifactorial satisfaction scale for primary care and mental health services. *Evaluation and Program Planning*, **12**, 271–278.

Greenfield, T. K. & Attkisson, C. C. (2000) Service Satisfaction Scale–30 (SSS–30). In *Handbook of Psychiatric Measures* (eds A. J. Rush, H. A. Pincus, M. B. First, *et al*), pp. 188–191. Washington, DC: American Psychiatric Association.

Greenfield, T. K. & Attkisson, C. C. (2004) The UCSF Client Satisfaction Scales: II. The Service Satisfaction Scale–30. In *Psychological Testing: Treatment Planning and Outcome Assessment. Vol. 3: Instruments for Adults* (ed. M. Maruish), pp. 813–837. Mahwah, NJ: Lawrence Erlbaum Associates.

Ruggeri, M. & Dall'Agnola, R. (1993) The development and use of the Verona Expectations for Care Scale (VECS) and the Verona Service Satisfaction Scale (VSSS) for measuring expectations and satisfaction with community-based psychiatruc services in patients, relatives and professionals. *Psychological Medicine*, **23**, 511–523.

Ruggeri, M., Dall'Agnola, R., Agostini, C., *et al* (1994) Acceptability, sensitivity and content validity of VECS and VSSS in measuring expectations and satisfaction in psychiatric patients and their relatives. *Social Psychiatry and Psychiatric Epidemiology*, **29**, 265–276.

Ruggeri, M. & Greenfield, T. (1995) The Italian version of the Service Satisfaction Scale (SSS–30) adapted for community-based psychiatric services: development, factor analysis and application. *Evaluation and Program Planning*, **18**, 191–202.

Ruggeri, M., Dall'Agnola, R., Bisoffi, G., *et al* (1996) Factor analysis of the Verona Satisfactin Scale–82 and development of reduced versions. *International Journal of Methods in Psychiatric Research*, **6**, 23–38.

Ruggeri, M., Lasalvia, A., Dall'Agnola, R., *et al* and the EPSILON Study Group (2000) Development, internal consistency and reliability of the Verona Satisfaction Scale – European Version. In *Reliable Outcome Measures for Mental Health Service Research in Five European Studies: The EPSILON Study* (eds G. Thornicroft, T. Becker, M. Knapp, *et al*). *British Journal of Psychiatry*, **177** (suppl. 39), 41–48.

Ruggeri, M., Lasalvia, A., Bisoffi, G., *et al* and the EPSILON Study Group (2003) Satisfaction with mental health services among people with schizophrenia in five European sites: results from the EPSILON Study. *Schizophrenia Bulletin*, **29**, 229–245.

17 Development and reliability of the VSSS–EU

*Mirella Ruggeri, Antonio Lasalvia, Rosa Dall'Agnola,
Bob van Wijngaarden, Helle Charlotte Knudsen,
Morven Leese, Andrés Herràn, Thomas Greenfield
and Michele Tansella*

Patient satisfaction is an important variable in the evaluation of psychiatric services and it complements the measurements of other outcome variables. It has been suggested (Kalman, 1983) that satisfaction is strictly linked to the effectiveness of the care provided, whereas dissatisfaction is frequently the reason behind patients' discontinuing psychiatric care (Ware *et al*, 1978; Hansen *et al*, 1992). Further, in cases where alternatives do not exist, as is often the case for people with serious mental disorders who may not be able to 'vote with their feet', it has been noted that assessment of satisfaction is crucial (Ruggeri & Greenfield, 1995). Ensuring high levels of patient satisfaction is, therefore, an essential aim for any mental health service, and its measurement constitutes a valid and important aspect of service planning and evaluation (Donabedian, 1966), to the extent that in many countries providers of health care are increasingly required to monitor levels of satisfaction among patients. Unfortunately, there is a lack of knowledge about the extent to which patients with psychosis are satisfied with services. This seems to be due both to prejudice against such patients, who are believed to be incapable of meaningfully judging the care they receive, and to methodological problems of measurement, mainly related to the difficulty of providing instruments that are acceptable to these patients.

Research in the area of satisfaction with psychiatric services has been hampered by the widespread use of many non-standardised methods, so that direct comparison between studies is usually impossible. Most studies have used instruments with few or no data regarding their validity or reliability, and investigators have frequently designed their own instruments for specific studies (Ruggeri & Greenfield, 1995). As a result, findings are not generalisable (Ruggeri, 1994). In addition, although satisfaction has been demonstrated to be a multi-dimensional concept (Ware *et al*, 1978; Greenfield & Attkisson, 1989), instruments have often been limited to a few broad items which only enquire about one or two dimensions of mental health care. Thus not only may they fail to detect any dissatisfaction – they are inherently unable to detect the reasons for dissatisfaction.

The Verona Service Satisfaction Scale (VSSS) (Ruggeri & Dall'Agnola, 1993) is a questionnaire meant to fill this gap: it is a validated, multi-dimensional scale which measures the satisfaction of patients with mental health services. First, an 82-item version was developed: it consisted of a set of 37 items relevant to a broad range of health services and a set of 45 items specific to mental health services. The former group of items involves aspects meant *a priori* to be relevant across a broad range of both medical and psychiatric settings, and was derived from the Service Satisfaction Scale (SSS–30) (Greenfield & Attkisson, 1989; Attkisson & Greenfield, 1994; Ruggeri & Greenfield, 1995). The latter group of items involves aspects that are specifically relevant in mental health settings, particularly in

146

community-based services, such as social skills and types of intervention (e.g. admissions, psychotherapy, rehabilitation) both newly developed and in some instances informed by derivative scales of the SSS for community- and hospital-based mental health programmes (for review see Greenfield & Attkisson, 2004). The 82-item VSSS, in its versions for patients and relatives, was tested for acceptability, content validity, sensitivity and test–retest reliability (Ruggeri & Dall'Agnola, 1993; Ruggeri *et al*, 1994) in 75 patients and 75 relatives. Finally, a factor analysis was performed (Ruggeri *et al*, 1996). The combination of results obtained in the validation study and factor analysis gave rise to the Intermediate (VSSS–54) and the Short (VSSS–32) versions, two reliable instruments that can be easily used in everyday clinical settings. The VSSS has been translated into various languages and used for research in many sites around the world; work already published concerns mainly the comparison between hospital- and community-based services (Parkman *et al*, 1997; Leese *et al*, 1998; Henderson *et al*, 1999). This chapter describes the development, translation, cultural validation and reliability of a new European version of the VSSS (VSSS–EU) for use in multi-site international comparative studies.

The EPSILON Study

The VSSS–EU was developed as part of the European Psychiatric Services: Inputs Linked to Outcome Domains and Needs (EPSILON) Study, being one of the mental health service research instruments to be produced in standardised forms in five European languages (Danish, Dutch, English, Italian and Spanish). The objectives of the study, the study sites and the populations surveyed are described in Chapter 1, and the methodology is discussed in Chapter 3.

Translation and adaptation

The VSSS–EU was developed from the Italian VSSS–54 version, following the translation procedure described in Chapter 2. Based on the progenitor SSS–30 series instruments, from which much item content and the measurement approach of the Verona scales derived, the VSSS–EU bears a strong similarity to the SSS–30 (Ruggeri & Greenfield, 1995; Attkisson & Greenfield, 1996; Greenfield & Attkisson, 2000) but also includes additional item content. The VSSS has been used largely in Europe, whereas the SSS has been widely used in the Americas, Australia and several other countries (Greenfield, 2000; Greenfield & Attkisson, 2004). The VSSS–54 was first translated into Danish, Dutch, English and Spanish by professional translators, and each translation was then back-translated into Italian. The back-translations were checked by the authors of the VSSS and compared with the original Italian version. (The English version of the VSSS–54 was compared with the SSS–30 by its American authors, with minor adjustments made to reduce unnecessary variation in wording between the English language instruments.) Small discrepancies in the VSSS were examined and alterations made to the Italian version in order to preserve the precise meaning of each question, while still producing an understandable and acceptable translation in the various languages. Specific items were changed to adapt them to the context of each country's mental health system; when such changes occurred, the local researchers made a list of the modifications. The next step was the focus group process, which discussed the content and the language of the translated instruments. In the light of the comments and recommendations, the instrument was then revised both in its original Italian version and in each of the four translations. On the basis of the focus groups' discussions, minor changes were made to the wording of the items, and a further change was made by deciding to make separate assessments of the skills and behaviour of psychiatrists, psychologists, nurses and social workers, rather than combining the professions into two groups as in the previous version. This innovation is unique to the VSSS–EU.

Conceptually, the items in the VSSS–EU cover seven dimensions: Overall Satisfaction, Professionals' Skills and Behaviour, Information, Access, Efficacy, Types of Intervention and Relative's Involvement. Items in the first five dimensions cover all areas belonging to Ware's taxonomy of satisfaction (Ware *et al*, 1983), also bearing a close relationship to three of four empirical satisfaction dimensions seen in the SSS–30: 'practitioner manner and skill', 'perceived outcome (efficacy)' and 'access' (Greenfield & Attkisson, 2004; and cf. Ruggeri & Greenfield, 1995). The last two VSSS–EU dimensions, on the other hand, examine domains that have not been assessed systematically in previous studies and have been specifically developed for the VSSS.

Each conceptual dimension of the VSSS–EU consists of a certain number of items that cover various aspects of satisfaction with services (Box 17.1):

(a)   the Overall Satisfaction dimension consists of three items which cover general aspects of satisfaction with psychiatric services;

(b)   the Professionals' Skills and Behaviour dimension consists of 24 items which cover various aspects of satisfaction with the professionals' behaviour, such as technical skills, interpersonal skills, cooperation between service providers and respect of patients' rights; psychiatrists, psychologists, nurses and social workers are assessed in separate items;

(c)   the Information dimension consists of three items which cover aspects related to satisfaction with information on services, disorders and therapies;

(d)   the Access dimension consists of two items which cover aspects related to satisfaction with service location, physical layout and costs;

(e)   the Efficacy dimension consists of eight items which cover aspects related to satisfaction with overall efficacy of the service, and service efficacy on specific aspects such as symptoms, social skills and family relationships;

(f)   the Types of Intervention dimension consists of 17 items which cover various aspects of satisfaction with care, such as drugs prescription, response to emergency, psychotherapy, rehabilitation, domiciliary care, admissions, housing, recreational activities, work and benefits;

(g)   the Relative's Involvement dimension consists of six items which cover various aspects of the patient's satisfaction with help given to his/her closest relative, such as listening, understanding, advice, information and help coping with the patient's problems.

The VSSS–EU is designed for self-administration and can be completed without prior training. In cases of cognitive deficit, severe psychopathologic disorder or low level of literacy, a research worker may assist the patient and/or the relative by reading through the items with them. Special care must be taken to guarantee confidentiality and anonymity and, in the case of assisted administration, to stress the independence of the research worker from the clinical team. Administering the questionnaire takes 20–30 minutes.

In the VSSS–EU, people are asked to express their overall feeling about their experience of the mental health service they have been using in the past year. For items 1–40, satisfaction ratings are on a five-point Likert scale (1 terrible, 2 mostly dissatisfied, 3 mixed, 4 mostly satisfied, 5 excellent), presented with alternate directionality to reduce stereotypic response. Items 41–54 consist of three questions: first, the respondent is asked if he or she has received the specific intervention ('Did you receive the intervention *x* in the past year?'). If the answer is 'yes', the person is asked to indicate his or her satisfaction on a 5-point Likert scale. If the answer is 'no', the person is asked 'Do you think you would have liked to receive intervention *x*?' (6 no, 7 don't know, 8 yes). These questions permit the estimation of the respondent's degree of satisfaction both with the interventions provided and with the professional's decision not to provide an intervention (if that was the case). The latter may be considered a measure of underprovision of care, from the patient's point of view.

Box 17.1   The seven dimensions of the VSSS–EU

Overall satisfaction (3 items)

11	Amount of help received
20	Kind of services
21	Overall satisfaction

Professionals' skills and behaviour (24 items)

3a	Professionalism and competence of the psychiatrists
3b	Professionalism and competence of the psychologists
16a	Thoroughness of psychiatrists
16b	Thoroughness of psychologists
22a	Professional competence of nursing staff
22b	Professional competence of social workers
35a	Thoroughness of nurses
35b	Thoroughness of social workers
6a	Psychiatrists' manner
6b	Psychologists' manner
5a	Ability of psychiatrists to listen and understand problems
5b	Ability of psychologists to listen and understand problems
25a	Nurses' manner
25b	Social workers' manner
28	Nurses' knowledge of patient's medical history
37a	Ability of nurses to listen and to understand problems
37b	Ability of social workers to listen and to understand problems
2	Behaviour and manners of reception or secretarial staff
33	Instruction on what to do between visits
18	Cooperation between service providers
17	Referring to general practitioner or other specialists
40	Opportunity of being followed up by the same professionals
10	Confidentiality and respect for patient's rights
7	Punctuality of the professionals when patient comes for an appointment

Information (3 items)

12	Explanation of specific procedures and approaches used
29	Information on diagnosis and prognosis
19	Publicity or information on mental health services which are offered

Access (2 items)

4	Appearance, comfort level and physical layout
8	Costs of the service

cont'd

Box 17.1   Continued

Efficacy (8 items)

9   Effectiveness of the service in attaining well-being and preventing relapses

1   Effectiveness of the service in helping patient deal with problems

24   Effectiveness of the service in helping patient improve knowledge and understanding of his/her
          problems

13   Effectiveness of the service in helping patient to relieve symptoms

26   Effectiveness of the service in improving the relationship between patient and relative

34   Effectiveness of the service in helping patient improve capacity to look after her/himself

31   Effectiveness of the service in helping patient establish good relationships outside family environment

38   Effectiveness of the service in helping patient improve abilities to work

Types of intervention (17 items)

14   Response of the service to crisis or urgent needs during office hours

15   Response of the service to emergencies during the night, weekends and public holidays

39   Help received for unexpected outcomes, discomfort or side-effects of medication

41   Medication prescription

42   Individual rehabilitation

43   Individual psychotherapy

44   Compulsory treatment in hospital

45   Family therapy

46   Living in sheltered accommodation

47   Participation in the recreational activities organised by mental health services

48   Group psychotherapy

49   Sheltered work

50   Informal admission to hospital

51   Practical help by the service at home

52   Help in obtaining welfare benefits or exemptions

53   Help to find open employment

54   Help from the service to join in recreational activities separate from the mental health services

Relative's involvement (6 items)

30a   Ability of psychiatrists to listen and understand the concerns and the opinions relative may have about
          patient

30b   Ability of psychologists to listen and understand the concerns and the opinions relative may have
          about patient

23   Recommendations about how relative could help

32   Information to relative about diagnosis and prognosis

36   Effectiveness of the service in helping relative to deal better with patient's problems

27   Effectiveness of the service in helping relative improve his/her understanding of patient's problems

Reliability assessment

Reliability testing in the EPSILON project was conducted on several levels, depending on the nature of the instruments involved and the way they were administered (interviews v. questionnaires). Details of the procedure are given in full in Chapter 3. As far as the VSSS–EU is concerned, the reliability tests were performed (a) on the VSSS–EU total mean score; (b) on the mean scores of each dimension; and (c) item by item, both for the pooled sample and across the five sites. Three kinds of reliability tests were used: Cronbach's α (Cronbach, 1951), to check the internal consistency of the whole questionnaire and the different dimensions; the intraclass correlation coefficient (ICC) (Bartko & Carpenter, 1976), to evaluate test–retest reliability of the VSSS–EU total mean score and dimension mean scores; and Cohen's weighted κ (Cohen, 1968), to evaluate test–retest reliability of single VSSS–EU items. Additional statistics estimated were the standard errors of measurement, which were obtained from the analysis of variance used to estimate the intraclass correlations.Statistical analysis was performed using SPSS for Windows, release 7.5 (Norusis, 1997), the Amsterdam α-testing program, ALPHA.EXE based on Feldt et al (1987) and EXCEL for tests of the homogeneity of ICCs.

A total sample of 289 participants (49 in Amsterdam, 43 in Copenhagen, 81 in London, 50 in Santander and 66 in Verona) completed both test and retest VSSS–EU administration. Retesting was done after a mean of 10.4 days (s.d. 6.03) in the pooled sample, 10.7 days (s.d. 7.45) in Amsterdam, 9.3 days (s.d. 3.57) in Copenhagen, 9.4 days (s.d. 3.93) in London, 6.1 days (s.d. 2.82) in Santander, 15.4 days (s.d. 6.70) in Verona. The shortest and longest test–retest intervals were in Santander and Verona, respectively (Kruskal–Wallis test, $P>0.001$).

Internal consistency

Table 17.1 shows the mean scores for each VSSS–EU dimension in the various EPSILON sites and the tests of homogeneity of variance (Levene test) and of means. Assuming that the standard error of measurement is the same in all countries, the reliability coefficient depends on the variance in each sample. Conversely, where standard errors of measurement do differ, sample variables will be affected, since they are composed both of variance in true scores and variation due to measurement error.

Table 17.1 Verona Service Satisfaction Scale – European Version sub-scales in the pooled sample and by site

Dimension	Pooled n=399 mean	s.d.	Amsterdam n=58 mean	s.d.	Copenhagen n=51 mean	s.d.	London n=83 mean	s.d.	Santander n=100 mean	s.d.	Verona n=107 mean	s.d.	Test of equality	Test of equality
Overall satisfaction	3.83	0.79	3.90	0.80	4.04	0.79	3.45	0.67	3.79	0.84	4.01	0.72	0.05	0.27
Professionals' skills and behaviour	3.88	0.57	3.97	0.51	4.13	0.56	3.46	0.40	3.94	0.53	4.00	0.60	<0.01	0.03
Information	3.39	0.93	3.66	0.75	3.69	0.86	3.26	0.65	2.93	1.09	3.64	0.88	<0.01	<0.01
Access	3.83	0.73	3.63	0.73	4.19	0.71	3.97	0.67	3.84	0.67	3.64	0.79	<0.01	0.35
Efficacy	3.56	0.74	3.69	0.69	3.80	0.76	3.22	0.55	3.41	0.77	3.81	0.74	<0.01	0.03
Types of intervention	3.64	0.42	3.65	0.47	3.72	0.42	3.68	0.24	3.42	0.41	3.75	0.46	<0.01	<0.01
Relative's involvement	3.39	0.96	3.57	0.92	3.32	1.21	2.91	0.67	3.39	0.96	3.75	0.91	<0.01	<0.01
Total score	3.70	0.50	3.79	0.46	3.89	0.48	3.45	0.34	3.59	0.51	3.96	0.54	<0.01	0.01

In all sites, sample sizes for each dimension varied slightly from the maximum: the number of cases dropped in each dimension was less than two, except in 'relative's involvement', for which the sample size was 359 in the pooled sample (49 in Amsterdam, 45 in Copenhagen, 80 in London, 96 in Santander and 89 in Verona).

Table 17.2 Internal consistency of the Verona Service Satisfaction Scale – European Version (VSSS–EU): α coefficients (95% CI) in the pooled sample and by site

Sub-scale	Items	Pooled sample		Amsterdam		Copenhagen		London		Santander		Verona		Test of equality
		n	α (95% CI)	n	α (95% CI)	n	α (95% CI)	n	α (95% CI)	n	α (95% CI)	n	α (95% CI)	P
Overall satisfaction	3	384	0.80 (0.77–0.83)	57	0.80 (0.71–0.87)	45	0.82 (0.73–0.88)	83	0.77 (0.69–0.83)	97	0.83 (0.78–0.88)	102	0.73 (0.65–0.80)	0.67
Professionals' skills and behaviour[1]	6	275	0.91 (0.89–0.92)	38	0.90 (0.89–0.95)	24	0.89 (0.82–0.95)	24	0.85 (0.80–0.89)	72	0.90 (0.86–0.93)	66	0.91 (0.88–0.94)	0.58
Information	3	342	0.72 (0.68–0.76)	51	0.67 (0.51–0.78)	40	0.60 (0.37–0.75)	82	0.63 (0.49–0.73)	72	0.79 (0.71–0.85)	97	0.72 (0.63–0.79)	0.39
Access	2	386	0.06 (−0.11 to 0.20)	53	0.16 (−0.33 to 0.47)	49	0.96 (0.93–0.97)	83	0.08 (−0.33 to 0.36)	99	0.77 (0.68–0.83)	102	0.29 (0.02–0.49)	<0.01
Efficacy	8	254	0.87 (0.84–0.87)	37	0.83 (0.75–0.89)	28	0.82 (0.73–0.90)	58	0.77 (0.68–0.84)	69	0.89 (0.85–0.92)	62	0.89 (0.85–0.92)	0.11
Types of intervention	17	115	0.73 (0.67–0.79)	19	0.81 (0.69–0.90)	8	0.61 (0.17–0.88)	52	0.62 (0.48–0.74)	4	–[2]	32	0.77 (0.66–0.86)	0.71
Relative's involvement	5	298	0.89 (0.87–0.91)	40	0.85 (0.77–0.91)	26	0.93 (0.88–0.97)	67	0.81 (0.72–0.87)	92	0.91 (0.87–0.94)	73	0.88 (0.82–0.91)	0.04
Total score	54	74	0.96 (0.94–0.97)	16	0.95 (0.91–0.98)	4	–[2]	33	0.93 (0.90–0.96)	2	–[2]	19	0.96 (0.93–0.98)	1.00

1. Three items were excluded from this analysis since they are utilised exclusively in specific situations ('if applicable'): for people married, retired or with previous hospitalisations.
2. Insufficient data to estimate α.

Therefore, when computing reliability coefficients and testing differences between samples, differences between sites in terms of both sample variance and standard errors of measurement should be considered.

The variability of the scores differed across the sites, both in the VSSS–EU total mean score and in all VSSS–EU dimensions, with the exception of Overall Satisfaction and Access; therefore the lack of homogeneity across the sites for the total mean scores and most of the dimension scores may account to some extent for the degree of variability in the reliability coefficients across the sites.

Table 17.2 shows the α coefficients and the test for the equality of α across the sites. Alpha coefficients indicate the degree to which items exhibit a positive correlation (internal consistency above 0.7 is considered adequate; Bech et al, 1993).

It should first be noted that the high degree of variability in the number of cases is usually not due to missing values but to the fact that some items (ability of psychologists to listen and understand the concerns and opinions relatives might have about the patients, thoroughness of psychologists, professionalism and competence of psychologists, thoroughness of social workers, professional competence of social workers, response of the service to emergencies during the night or at weekends) are not applicable to all patients. For this reason, α values in the VSSS–EU total mean scores have been computed for a small number of cases only. However, they were always over 0.90 and were similar across the sites, with the exception of Relative's Involvement. In the VSSS–EU dimensions, α coefficients ranged from 0.60 (Information dimension, in Copenhagen) to 0.93 (Relative's Involvement dimension, in Copenhagen) and did not differ significantly across the sites. The dimension Access, which consists of just two items (Costs of Service and Physical Layout) measuring different constructs, is a special case. In this dimension, α varied greatly, ranging from 0.08 (London) to 0.96 (Copenhagen), and differed significantly across the sites. Dimensions constituted by a higher number of items are expected to have higher α values. This was true for the dimension Professionals' Skills and Behaviour, but not for the dimension Types of Intervention, which is not expected to have high internal consistency, owing to the wide range of different interventions explored by the questionnaire.

On the whole, α values of the pooled sample were good, with the above-mentioned exception of the Access dimension, and ranged from 0.72 (Information) to 0.91 (Professionals' Skills and Behaviour).

Stability

The test–retest reliability was studied by considering the ratings both in each dimension (ICC) and item by item (weighted κ). Table 17.3 shows the test–retest reliability for the VSSS–EU total mean score and VSSS–EU dimension scores, both in the pooled sample and at each EPSILON site. Intraclass correlation coefficients and the standard errors of measurements are reported. The VSSS–EU total mean score in the pooled sample shows a high degree of reliability (0.82; 95% CI 0.78–0.85), although there are some differences between the sites, with all sites above 0.70 and three sites (Copenhagen, London and Santander) above 0.80. Each of the VSSS–EU dimension mean scores in the pooled sample had a degree of reliability ranging from 0.56 to 0.78. The reliability of the VSSS–EU dimension mean scores across the sites was over 0.50 in all cases, with the exception of the Access dimension in Santander (0.43) and the Information dimension in Amsterdam (0.49). Overall, there was some degree of variability in the ICC coefficients across the sites. This could be due either to differences in measurement errors between different sites, or to lack of homogeneity in the samples. The lower reliabilities tend to be associated with higher standard errors of measurement, and therefore lack of homogeneity in the samples is unlikely to be the explanation for differences in reliability; rather, the performance of the instrument itself differs.

Table 17.4 shows Cohen's weighted κ for both the pooled sample and the five EPSILON sites, calculated in each VSSS–EU item by taking the disagreements' weight to be equal to the square of the

Table 17.3 Test–retest reliability of the Verona Service Satisfaction Scale – European Version dimensions and total mean scores in the pooled sample and by site

Sub-scale	Pooled n=289		Amsterdam n=49		Copenhagen n=43		London n=81		Santander n=50		Verona n=66		Test of equality of ICCs (P)
	ICC	(s.e.)$_m$	ICC	(s.e.)$_m$	ICC	(s.e.)$_m$	ICC	(s.e.)$_m$	ICC	(s.e.)$_m$	ICC	(s.e.)$_m$	
Overall satisfaction	0.66	0.44	0.50	0.51	0.67	0.46	0.76	0.33	0.80	0.37	0.52	0.52	0.01
Professionals' skills and behaviour	0.76	0.25	0.66	0.29	0.80	0.24	0.78	0.19	0.86	0.19	0.72	0.31	0.06
Information	0.75	0.14	0.49	0.52	0.75	0.42	0.66	0.37	0.84	0.44	0.76	0.41	<0.01
Access	0.56	0.47	0.56	0.48	0.51	0.49	0.73	0.33	0.43	0.51	0.51	0.55	0.05
Efficacy	0.75	0.34	0.70	0.36	0.76	0.35	0.77	0.26	0.90	0.23	0.59	0.45	<0.01
Types of intervention	0.69	0.22	0.56	0.32	0.64	0.25	0.82	0.09	0.90	0.13	0.66	0.26	<0.01
Relative's involvement	0.78	0.43	0.72	0.47	0.82	0.53	0.70	0.38	0.89	0.32	0.67	0.48	<0.01
Total score	0.82	0.20	0.73	0.24	0.85	0.19	0.82	0.15	0.93	0.13	0.76	0.25	<0.01

ICC, intraclass correlation coefficient; (s.e.)$_m$, standard error of measurement (square root of error components of variance).

distances. According to Landis & Koch (1977), a κ coefficient of 0.2–0.4 indicates fair agreement, 0.4–0.6 indicates moderate agreement, 0.6–0.8 indicates a substantial agreement and 0.8–1.0 indicates almost perfect agreement, although alternative schemes are possible (see Chapter 3).

In the pooled sample, all items generated κ coefficients from 0.4 to 0.8, indicating a moderate to substantial agreement. In the various EPSILON sites the percentage of items with κ coefficients exceeding 0.4 (generally accepted as the minimum value) ranged from 54% (Verona) to 97% (London).

A paired sample *t*-test on the difference between test and retest for the VSSS–EU total mean scores and dimension sub-scores revealed no significant differences, both pooled across sites and at individual sites (with the exception of Access in London and Santander, where the retest values were respectively higher and lower than the time 1 values, *P*<0.001), thus showing no overall tendency for patients to respond more or less favourably after an interval ranging from 1 week to 2 weeks.

Discussion

Although there is little doubt that patient satisfaction is an important aspect in the assessment of the quality and outcome of community-based mental health programmes, research suffers from various methodological limitations regarding study design, the construction of the instrument and the lack of

Table 17.4 Test–retest reliability of individual items of the Verona Service Satisfaction Scale – European Version: number (percentage) of items in Cohen's weighted κ bands

Weighted κ	Strength of agreement	Pooled n=26 n (%)	Amsterdam n=49 n (%)	Copenhagen n=43 n (%)	London n=81 n (%)	Santander n=50 n (%)	Verona n=66 n (%)
0.81–1.0	Almost perfect			2 (3)	14 (22)	10 (16)	
0.61–0.80	Substantial	31 (49)	8 (13)	23 (36)	36 (57)	33 (52)	8 (12.7)
0.41–0.60	Moderate	32 (51)	37 (59)	25 (40)	11 (17)	16 (25)	26 (41.2)
0.21–0.40	Fair		18 (29)	10 (16)	2 (3)	4 (6)	22 (34.9)
0–0.20	Slight			3 (5)			7 (11.1)

Weighted κ bands suggested by Landis & Koch (1977).

attention to its psychometric properties. According to many authors, the lack of attention to methodological aspects and the lack of confidentiality strongly influence levels of reported satisfaction (Larsen *et al*, 1979; Weinstein, 1979; Keppler-Seid *et al*, 1980; Ruggeri, 1994). One of the most important aims during the development of the original version of the VSSS was the avoidance of methodological biases: data previously obtained on content validity, test–retest reliability and factor analysis showed that the original version measured satisfaction in a sensitive, valid and reliable way (Ruggeri & Dall'Agnola, 1993; Ruggeri *et al*, 1994, 1996). The newly developed VSSS–EU has now also been shown to have good psychometric properties.

The scale has an excellent overall Cronbach's α (0.96), which confirms its adequacy from the standpoint of internal consistency if it is used as a global satisfaction measure. All dimensions except one (Access) showed good internal consistency, as indicated by α values ranging from 0.72 for Information to 0.91 for Professionals' Skills and Behaviour. The dimension with the lowest consistency (Access), made up of two items (Cost of Service and Physical Layout), was not expected to show high interrelatedness, because theoretically these two items are independent of one another.

The test–retest data provided encouraging results. The stability of the scale was satisfactory both at dimensional level and item by item. Although there was some evidence of differences in reliability between sites, which was associated with different standard errors of measurement rather than different homogeneity of the samples, all the individual site reliability coefficients for the total score were above 0.7. Interestingly, the lowest test–retest reliability was found in Verona, thus indicating that the translation of the scale did not affect its acceptability to patients. The overall pooled test–retest reliability for the total score was excellent at 0.82 (95% CI 0.78–0.85). Furthermore, there was no evidence of any tendency for the measurements to change systematically over time, either in the pooled sample or across the sites (with the above-mentioned exception of Access).

In conclusion, the analysis of the data presented here demonstrates that the VSSS–EU has good psychometric properties and suggests that it is a reliable instrument for measuring satisfaction with mental health services in people with schizophrenia, for use in comparative cross-national research projects and in routine clinical practice in mental health services across Europe.

References and further reading

Attkisson, C. C. & Greenfield, T. K. (1994) The Client Satisfaction Questionnaire–8 and the Services Satisfaction Questionnaire–30. In *Psychological Testing: Treatment Planning and Outcome Assessment* (ed. M. Maruish), pp. 404–420. San Francisco: Lawrence Erlbaum Associates.

Attkisson, C. C. & Greenfield, T. K. (1996) The Client Satisfaction Questionnaire (CSQ) scales and the Service Satisfaction Scale–30 (SSS–30). In *Outcomes Assessment in Clinical Practice* (eds L. I. Sederer & B. Dickey), pp. 120–127. Baltimore, MD: Williams & Wilkins.

Bartko, J. J. & Carpenter, W. T. (1976) On the methods and theory of reliability. *Journal of Nervous and Mental Disease*, **163**, 307–317.

Bech, P., Mault, U. F., Dencker, S. J., *et al* (1993) Scales for assessment of diagnosis and severity of mental disorders. *Acta Psychiatrica Scandinavica*, **87** (suppl. 372), 1–87.

Cohen, J. (1968) Weighted kappa: nominal scale agreement with provision for scaled disagreement or partial credit. *Psychological Bulletin*, **70**, 213–220.

Cronbach, L. J. (1951) Coefficient alpha and the internal structure of tests. *Psychometrika*, **16**, 297–334.

Donabedian, A. (1966) Evaluating the quality of medical care. *Millbank Memorial Fund Quarterly*, **44**, 166–203.

Feldt, L. S., Woodruff, D. J. & Salih, F. A. (1987) Statistical inference for coefficient alpha. *Applied Psychological Measurement*, **11**, 93–103.

Greenfield, T. K. (2000) Case examples of client satisfaction evaluations: Parts A and B. In *WHO Evaluation of Psychoactive Substance Use Disorder Treatment, Workbook 6: Client Satisfaction Evaluations* (ed. M. Monteiro), pp. 21–31. Geneva: WHO, Substance Abuse Department. http://whqlibdoc.who.int/hq/2000/WHO_MSD_MSB_00.2g.pdf

Greenfield, T. K. & Attkisson, C. C. (1989) Steps toward a multifactorial satisfaction scale for primary care and mental health services. *Evaluation and Program Planning*, **12**, 271–278.

Greenfield, T. K. & Attkisson, C. C. (2000) Service Satisfaction Scale–30 (SSS–30). In *Handbook of Psychiatric Measures* (eds A. J. Rush, H. A. Pincus, M. B. First, *et al*), pp. 188–191. Washington, DC: American Psychiatric Association.

Greenfield, T. K. & Attkisson, C. C. (2004) The UCSF Client Satisfaction Scales: II. The Service Satisfaction Scale–30. In *Psychological Testing: Treatment Planning and Outcome Assessment. Vol. 3: Instruments for Adults* (ed. M. Maruish), pp. 813–837. Mahwah, NJ: Lawrence Erlbaum Associates.

Hansen, A. M. D., Hoogduin, C. A. L., Schaap, C., *et al* (1992) Do dropouts differ from successfully treated obsessive-compulsives? *Behavioural Research and Therapy*, **30**, 547–550.

Henderson, C., Phelan, M., Loftus, L., *et al* (1999) Comparison of patient satisfaction with community-based vs. hospital psychiatric services. *Acta Psychiatrica Scandinavica*, **99**, 188–195.

Kalman, T. P. (1983) An overview of patient satisfaction with psychiatric treatment. *Hospital and Community Psychiatry*, **34**, 48–54.

Keppler-Seid, H., Windle, C. & Woy, J. (1980) Performance measures for mental health programs. *Community Mental Health Journal*, **16**, 217–234.

Landis, J. & Koch, G. (1977) The measurement of the observer agreement for categorical data. *Biometrics*, **33**, 159–174.

Larsen, D. L., Attkisson, C. C., Hargreaves, W. A., *et al* (1979) Assessment of client/patients' satisfaction: development of a general scale. *Evaluation and Program Planning*, **2**, 197–207.

Leese, M., Johnson, S., Slade, M., *et al* (1998) User perspective on needs and satisfaction with mental health services. PRiSM Psychosis Study 8. *British Journal of Psychiatry*, **173**, 409–415.

Norusis, G. (1997) *Statistical Package for Social Sciences (SPSS). Release 7.5*. Chicago, IL: SPSS Inc.

Parkman, S., Davies S., Leese, M., *et al* (1997) Ethnic differences in satisfaction with mental health services among representative people with psychosis in South London: PRiSM Study 4. *British Journal of Psychiatry*, **171**, 260–264.

Ruggeri, M. (1994) Patients' and relatives' satisfaction with psychiatric services: the state of the art of its measurement. *Social Psychiatry and Psychiatric Epidemiology*, **28**, 212–227.

Ruggeri, M. & Dall'Agnola, R. (1993) The development and use of the Verona Expectations for Care Scale (VECS) and the Verona Service Satisfaction Scale (VSSS) for measuring expectations and satisfaction with community-based psychiatric services in patients, relatives and professionals. *Psychological Medicine*, **23**, 511–523.

Ruggeri, M. & Greenfield, T. (1995) The Italian version of the Service Satisfaction Scale (SSS–30) adapted for community-based psychiatric services: development, factor analysis and application. *Evaluation and Program Planning*, **18**, 191–202.

Ruggeri, M., Dall'Agnola, R., Agostini, C., *et al* (1994) Acceptability, sensitivity and content validity of VECS and VSSS in measuring expectations and satisfaction in psychiatric patients and their relatives. *Social Psychiatry and Psychiatric Epidemiology*, **29**, 265–276.

Ruggeri, M., Dall'Agnola, R., Bisoffi, G., *et al* (1996) Factor analysis of the Verona Service Satisfaction Scale–82 and development of reduced versions. *International Journal of Methods in Psychiatric Research*, **6**, 23–38.

Ware, J. E., Davies-Avery, A. & Stewart, A. (1978) The measurement and meaning of patient satisfaction: a review of the recent literature. *Health and Medical Care Services Review*, **1**, 1–15.

Ware, J. E., Snyder, M. K., Wright, W. R., *et al* (1983) Defining and measuring patient satisfaction with medical care. *Evaluation and Program Planning*, **6**, 247–263.

Weinstein, R. (1979) Patient attitudes toward mental hospitals. *Journal of Health and Social Behaviour*, **20**, 237–258.

World Health Organization (1992) *Schedules for Clinical Assessment in Neuropsychiatry* (ed.-in-chief J. K. Wing). Geneva: WHO.

18 Verona Service Satisfaction Scale – European Version

Mirella Ruggeri, Thomas Greenfield and Rosa Dall'Agnola

The Verona Satisfaction Scale – European Version for Patients (VSSS–EU)[1,2]

Introduction

This questionnaire asks about your experience of the community mental health services offered locally, during the past year.

It is very important that you answer **truthfully**; please express your opinion **whatever it is**. We are especially interested to know about your **criticisms** and about **problems** you might have had with the services.

All your answers will be treated **confidentially**. They will not be discussed with the professionals working in the service or your relatives.

Please feel free to ask the researcher for help if a question is not clear or if you encounter any problem in filling in the questionnaire.

Please read the instructions very carefully and take your time before answering. It is very important that every answer expresses your true opinion.

In the following pages, we ask you about your experiences in using the local mental health services during the past year.

Please mark the answer that best describes your overall impression in using the local mental health services during the past year.

You can use one of these options:

1. Terrible
2. Mostly <u>dis</u>satisfied
3. Mixed
4. Mostly satisfied
5. Excellent

Please choose the answer that is the best description of your experience in using the local mental health services over the **past year**:

What is your overall feeling about the:

1. **effect of services in helping you to deal with your problems?**

    1. Terrible   2. Mostly   3. Mixed   4. Mostly   5. Excellent
                     dissatisfied   satisfied

2. **behaviour and manners of reception or secretarial staff on the telephone or when you meet them?**

    5. Excellent   4. Mostly   3. Mixed   2. Mostly   1. Terrible
                     satisfied   dissatisfied

3a. **professional knowledge and competence of *psychiatrists***

    1. Terrible   2. Mostly   3. Mixed   4. Mostly   5. Excellent
                     dissatisfied   satisfied

3b. **professional knowledge and competence of *psychologists***

    5. Excellent   4. Mostly   3. Mixed   2. Mostly   1. Terrible
                     satisfied   dissatisfied

4. **the appearance, comfort level and physical layout of the facilities**
    (e.g. the waiting rooms and the offices)

    1. Terrible   2. Mostly   3. Mixed   4. Mostly   5. Excellent
                     dissatisfied   satisfied

5a. **ability of psychiatrists to listen and to understand your problems**

    5. Excellent   4. Mostly   3. Mixed   2. Mostly   1. Terrible
                     satisfied   dissatisfied

5b. **ability of psychologists to listen and to understand your problems**

    1. Terrible   2. Mostly   3. Mixed   4. Mostly   5. Excellent
                     dissatisfied   satisfied

6a. **personal manner of *psychiatrists***

    5. Excellent   4. Mostly   3. Mixed   2. Mostly   1. Terrible
                     satisfied   dissatisfied

6b. **personal manner of *psychologists***

    1. Terrible   2. Mostly   3. Mixed   4. Mostly   5. Excellent
                     dissatisfied   satisfied

7. **punctuality of the professionals when you come for an appointment**

    5. Excellent   4. Mostly   3. Mixed   2. Mostly   1. Terrible
                     satisfied   dissatisfied

Please read the questions very carefully and take your time before answering.
It is very important that every answer expresses your true opinion.

8.   cost of the service to you (e.g. prescription charges)

1. Terrible   2. Mostly   3. Mixed   4. Mostly   5. Excellent
                        dissatisfied   satisfied

9.   effectiveness of services in helping you to attain well-being and preventing relapse

5. Excellent   4. Mostly   3. Mixed   2. Mostly   1. Terrible
                        satisfied   dissatisfied

10.   confidentiality and respect for your rights

1. Terrible   2. Mostly   3. Mixed   4. Mostly   5. Excellent
                        dissatisfied   satisfied

11.   amount of help you have received

5. Excellent   4. Mostly   3. Mixed   2. Mostly   1. Terrible
                        satisfied   dissatisfied

12.   explanations of specific procedures or approaches used

1. Terrible   2. Mostly   3. Mixed   4. Mostly   5. Excellent
                        dissatisfied   satisfied

13.   effect of services in helping to relieve symptoms

5. Excellent   4. Mostly   3. Mixed   2. Mostly   1. Terrible
                        satisfied   dissatisfied

14.   response of the service to crises or urgent needs during office hours

1. Terrible   2. Mostly   3. Mixed   4. Mostly   5. Excellent
                        dissatisfied   satisfied

15.   arrangements made for after hours emergencies

5. Excellent   4. Mostly   3. Mixed   2. Mostly   1. Terrible
                        satisfied   dissatisfied

16a.   thoroughness of psychiatrists

1. Terrible   2. Mostly   3. Mixed   4. Mostly   5. Excellent
                        dissatisfied   satisfied

16b.   thoroughness of psychologists

5. Excellent   4. Mostly   3. Mixed   2. Mostly   1. Terrible
                        satisfied   dissatisfied

17.   appropriateness of referrals to your GP or other specialist if needed

1. Terrible   2. Mostly   3. Mixed   4. Mostly   5. Excellent
                        dissatisfied   satisfied

18.   cooperation between service providers (if you are treated by more than one professional)

5. Excellent   4. Mostly   3. Mixed   2. Mostly   1. Terrible
                        satisfied   dissatisfied

Please read the questions very carefully and take your time before answering.
It is very important that every answer expresses your true opinion.

19. **publicity or information about available mental health services**

    1. Terrible   2. Mostly dissatisfied   3. Mixed   4. Mostly satisfied   5. Excellent

20. **kinds of service offered**

    5. Excellent   4. Mostly satisfied   3. Mixed   2. Mostly dissatisfied   1. Terrible

21. **in an overall, general sense, the service you have received**

    1. Terrible   2. Mostly dissatisfied   3. Mixed   4. Mostly satisfied   5. Excellent

22a. **professional knowledge and competence of *nurses***

    5. Excellent   4. Mostly satisfied   3. Mixed   2. Mostly dissatisfied   1. Terrible

22b. **professional knowledge and competence of *social workers***

    1. Terrible   2. Mostly dissatisfied   3. Mixed   4. Mostly satisfied   5. Excellent

23. **recommendations made to your closest relative about how they could help you**

    5. Excellent   4. Mostly satisfied   3. Mixed   2. Mostly dissatisfied   1. Terrible

24. **effectiveness of the service in helping you to improve your knowledge and understanding of your problems**

    1. Terrible   2. Mostly dissatisfied   3. Mixed   4. Mostly satisfied   5. Excellent

25a. **personal manners of *nurses***

    5. Excellent   4. Mostly satisfied   3. Mixed   2. Mostly dissatisfied   1. Terrible

25b. **personal manners of social workers**

    1. Terrible   2. Mostly dissatisfied   3. Mixed   4. Mostly satisfied   5. Excellent

26. **effectiveness of the service in improving the relationship between you and your closest relative**

    5. Excellent   4. Mostly satisfied   3. Mixed   2. Mostly dissatisfied   1. Terrible

27. **effectiveness of the service in helping your main carer (relative or friend) improve their understanding of your problems**

    1. Terrible   2. Mostly dissatisfied   3. Mixed   4. Mostly satisfied   5. Excellent

Please read the questions very carefully and take your time before answering.
It is very important that every answer expresses your true opinion.

Please choose the answer that is the best description of your experience in using the local mental health services over the **past year**:

What is your overall feeling about the:

28. nurses' knowledge about you and your medical history

5. Excellent	4. Mostly satisfied	3. Mixed	2. Mostly dissatisfied	1. Terrible

29. how information was given to you about your problem (diagnosis) and what to expect (prognosis)

1. Terrible	2. Mostly dissatisfied	3. Mixed	4. Mostly satisfied	5. Excellent

30a. ability of *psychiatrists* to listen and understand the worries your main carer (relative or friend) may have about you

5. Excellent	4. Mostly satisfied	3. Mixed	2. Mostly dissatisfied	1. Terrible

30b. ability of *psychologists* to listen and to understand the worries your main carer (relative or friend) may have about you

1. Terrible	2. Mostly dissatisfied	3. Mixed	4. Mostly satisfied	5. Excellent

31. effectiveness of the service in helping you establish good relationships with people outside your family (e.g. friends, neighbours, colleagues at work, etc.)

5. Excellent	4. Mostly satisfied	3. Mixed	2. Mostly dissatisfied	1. Terrible

32. how information was given to your main carer (relative or friend) about your problem (diagnosis) and what to expect (prognosis)

1. Terrible	2. Mostly dissatisfied	3. Mixed	4. Mostly satisfied	5. Excellent

33. instructions about what to do on your own between appointments; the clarity, practicality, etc. of recommendations

5. Excellent	4. Mostly satisfied	3. Mixed	2. Mostly dissatisfied	1. Terrible

34. effectiveness of the service in helping you to improve your self-care (e.g. taking care of your personal hygiene, your diet, your room)

1. Terrible	2. Mostly dissatisfied	3. Mixed	4. Mostly satisfied	5. Excellent

Please read the questions very carefully and take your time before answering.
It is very important that every answer expresses your true opinion.

Please choose the answer that is the best description of your experience in using the local mental health services over the **past year**:

What is your overall feeling about the:

35a. thoroughness of *nurses*

5. Excellent   4. Mostly   3. Mixed   2. Mostly   1. Terrible
                   satisfied   dissatisfied

35b. thoroughness of *social workers*

1. Terrible   2. Mostly   3. Mixed   4. Mostly   5. Excellent
                   dissatisfied   satisfied

36.   effectiveness of the service in helping your main carer (relative or friend) deal better with your problems

5. Excellent   4. Mostly   3. Mixed   2. Mostly   1. Terrible
                   satisfied   dissatisfied

37a. ability of *nurses* to listen to and understand your problems

1. Terrible   2. Mostly   3. Mixed   4. Mostly   5. Excellent
                   dissatisfied   satisfied

37b. ability of *social workers* to listen to and understand your problems

5. Excellent   4. Mostly   3. Mixed   2. Mostly   1. Terrible
                   satisfied   dissatisfied

38.   effectiveness of the service in helping you to improve your ability to work

1. Terrible   2. Mostly   3. Mixed   4. Mostly   5. Excellent
                   dissatisfied   satisfied

39.   help you have received for side-effects from medications (if occurred)

5. Excellent   4. Mostly   3. Mixed   2. Mostly   1. Terrible
                   satisfied   dissatisfied

40.   continuity of care (seeing the same staff) you have received

1. Terrible   2. Mostly   3. Mixed   4. Mostly   5. Excellent
                   dissatisfied   satisfied

Please read the questions very carefully and take your time before answering.
It is very important that every answer expresses your true opinion.

Please choose the answer that is the best description of your experience in using the local mental health services over the **past year**:

41. **In the past year, have you been prescribed medication?** (Please choose YES or NO)

YES
If you have answered YES, what is your overall feeling about this/them?

1. Terrible   2. Mostly   3. Mixed   4. Mostly   5. Excellent
                        unsatisfactory   satisfactory

NO
If you have answered NO, do you think you would have liked to receive this/them?

6. No   7. Don't know   8. Yes

42. **In the past year, did you receive help from staff to improve your capacity to cope with your social and working life?** (e.g. going to public offices, doing housework, getting on with your family and others) (Please choose YES or NO)

YES
If you have answered YES, what is your overall feeling about this/them?

5. Excellent   4. Mostly   3. Mixed   2. Mostly   1. Terrible
                        satisfactory   unsatisfactory

NO
If you have answered NO, do you think you would have liked to receive this?

6. No   7. Don't know   8. Yes

43. **In the past year, did you have the opportunity to meet alone, on a regular basis, with your therapist?** (e.g. in order to help you understand your problems and/or change your behaviour in some way) (Please choose YES or NO)

YES
If you have answered YES, what is your overall feeling about this/them?

1. Terrible   2. Mostly   3. Mixed   4. Mostly   5. Excellent
                        unsatisfactory   satisfactory

NO
If you have answered NO, do you think you would have liked to receive this?

6. No   7. Don't know   8. Yes

Please read the questions very carefully and take your time before answering.
It is very important that every answer expresses your true opinion.

Please choose the answer that is the best description of your experience in using the local mental health services over the **past year**:

44. **In the past year, did you have compulsory treatment in a psychiatric hospital?**
     (Please choose YES or NO)

     YES
     If you have answered YES, what is your overall feeling about this/them?

     5. Excellent   4. Mostly   3. Mixed   2. Mostly   1. Terrible
                         satisfactory   unsatisfactory

     NO
     If you have answered NO, do you think you would have liked to receive this?

     6. No   7. Don't know   8. Yes

45. **In the past year, did you have meetings with your family and therapist?** (with the aim
     of improving/changing the relationships between family members) (Please choose YES or NO)

     YES
     If you have answered YES, what is your overall feeling about this/them?

     1. Terrible   2. Mostly   3. Mixed   4. Mostly   5. Excellent
                         unsatisfactory   satisfactory

     NO
     If you have answered NO, do you think you would have liked to receive this/them?

     6. No   7. Don't know   8. Yes

46. **In the past year, did you have a place in sheltered accommodation?** (e.g. foster
     home/family placement scheme, group home, hostel with staff available for help)
     (Please choose YES or NO)

     YES
     If you have answered YES, what is your overall feeling about this/them?

     5. Excellent   4. Mostly   3. Mixed   2. Mostly   1. Terrible
                         satisfactory   unsatisfactory

     NO
     If you have answered NO, do you think you would have liked to receive this?

     6. No   7. Don't know   8. Yes

*Please read the questions very carefully and take your time before answering.
It is very important that every answer expresses your true opinion.*

Please choose the answer that is the best description of your experience in using the local mental health services over the **past year**:

47. **In the past year, did you have the opportunity to take part in leisure activities organised by the mental health services?** (Please choose YES or NO)

    YES
    If you have answered YES, what is your overall feeling about this/them?

1. Terrible	2. Mostly unsatisfactory	3. Mixed	4. Mostly satisfactory	5. Excellent

    NO
    If you have answered NO, do you think you would have liked to receive this/them?

    6. No   7. Don't know   8. Yes

48. **In the past year, did you have group psychotherapy?** (e.g. meetings of a group of patients with one or more therapists with the aim of improving the patient's understanding of their problems and/or changing their behaviour) (Please choose YES or NO)

    YES
    If you have answered YES, what is your overall feeling about this/them?

5. Excellent	4. Mostly satisfactory	3. Mixed	2. Mostly unsatisfactory	1. Terrible

    NO
    If you have answered NO, do you think you would have liked to receive this?

    6. No   7. Don't know   8. Yes

49. **In the past year, did you have any sheltered work?** (Please choose YES or NO)

    YES
    If you have answered YES, what is your overall feeling about this?

1. Terrible	2. Mostly unsatisfactory	3. Mixed	4. Mostly satisfactory	5. Excellent

    NO
    If you have answered NO, do you think you would have liked to receive this?

    6. No   7. Don't know   8. Yes

Please read the questions very carefully and take your time before answering.
It is very important that every answer expresses your true opinion.

Please choose the answer that is the best description of your experience in using the local mental health services over the **past year**:

50. **In the past year, did you have any voluntary admissions to a psychiatric hospital?** (Please choose YES or NO)

YES
If you have answered YES, what is your overall feeling about this/them?

5. Excellent	4. Mostly satisfactory	3. Mixed	2. Mostly unsatisfactory	1. Terrible

NO
If you have answered NO, do you think you would have liked to receive this/them?

6. No   7. Don't know   8. Yes

51. **In the past year, did you have practical help at home from the service?** (e.g. companionship, home help, etc.) (Please choose YES or NO)

YES
If you have answered YES, what is your overall feeling about this?

1. Terrible	2. Mostly unsatisfactory	3. Mixed	4. Mostly satisfactory	5. Excellent

NO
If you have answered NO, do you think you would have liked to receive this?

6. No   7. Don't know   8. Yes

52. **In the past year, did you have help from the service obtaining welfare benefits or exemptions?** (e.g. Disability Allowance, Council Tax, etc.) (Please choose YES or NO)

YES
If you have answered YES, what is your overall feeling about this?

5. Excellent	4. Mostly satisfactory	3. Mixed	2. Mostly unsatisfactory	1. Terrible

NO
If you have answered NO, do you think you would have liked to receive this?

6. No   7. Don't know   8. Yes

Please read the questions very carefully and take your time before answering.
It is very important that every answer expresses your true opinion.

Please choose the answer that is the best description of your experience in using the local mental health services over the **past year**:

53. **In the past year, did you have help from the service finding open employment?**
(Please choose YES or NO)

YES
If you have answered YES, what is your overall feeling about this?

1. Terrible	2. Mostly unsatisfactory	3. Mixed	4. Mostly satisfactory	5. Excellent

NO
If you have answered NO, do you think you would have liked to receive this?

6. No   7. Don't know   8. Yes

54. **In the past year, did you receive help from the services to join in leisure activities separate from the mental health services?** (Please choose YES or NO)

YES
If you have answered YES, what is your overall feeling about this?

5. Excellent	4. Mostly satisfactory	3. Mixed	2. Mostly unsatisfactory	1. Terrible

NO
If you have answered NO, do you think you would have liked to receive this?

6. No   7. Don't know   8. Yes

Please read the questions very carefully and take your time before answering.
It is very important that every answer expresses your true opinion.

Please write your comments:

The thing that I have liked most about my experience of mental health services is:

_____
_____
_____
_____
_____
_____
_____
_____
_____
_____

The thing that I have disliked most about my experience of local mental health services is:

_____
_____
_____
_____
_____
_____
_____
_____
_____
_____
_____
_____

Thank you very much for your help

Notes and copyright information
1. Ruggeri M. & Dall'Agnola R. (1993) The development and use of the Verona Expectations for Care Scale (VECS) and the Verona Service Satisfaction Scale (VSSS) for measuring expectations and satisfaction with community-based psychiatric services in patients, relatives and professionals. *Psychological Medicine*, **23**, 511–523.
   Numerous items and the scale's format were adopted, translated (and back-translated) or adapted, with permission of the authors (Greenfield, Attkisson & Pascoe), from the Service Satisfaction Scale–30 or derived instruments (Greenfield, T. K. & Attkisson, C. C. (1989) Steps toward a multifactorial satisfaction scale for primary care and mental health services. *Evaluation and Program Planning*, **12**, 271–278). For detailed list see Ruggeri, M. & Greenfield, T. K. (1995) The Italian version of the Service Satisfaction Scale (SSS 30) adapted for community-based psychiatric services. *Evaluation and Program Planning*, **18**, 191–202.
2. Ruggeri, M., Lasalvia A., Dall'Agnola R, *et al* (2000) Development, internal consistency and reliability of the Verona Service Satisfaction Scale – European Version. EPSILON Study 7. *British Journal of Psychiatry*, **177** (suppl. 39), 41–48.

Index

Compiled by Linda English